M000046338

COVID 19

PANDEMIC OF FEAR

Are medical and scientific facts being obscured by politics?

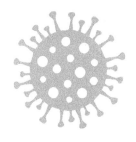

MARGARET STEVENSON

The COVID-19 Pandemic of Fear by Margaret Stevenson
Published by Publish My Book Online
www.publishmybook.online
Copyright 2021 © Margaret Stevenson
www.margaretstevenson.com.au

The information in this book is not intended to be utilised by
anyone as direct medical advice. Its only purpose is to make the
reader aware of documented scientific information and other
treatment possibilities that can be discussed further with a
chosen health care professional.
Statements made in this book should be regarded as my own
submitted for the reader's scrutiny and should not be attributed
to any person or persons named herein.

Scripture quotations are from The Holy Bible, English Standard
Version® (ESV®), copyright © 2001 by Crossway, a publishing
ministry of Good News Publishers. Used by permission.
All rights reserved.

1st Edition 2021
ISBN: 978-1-925999-98-3   paperback
ISBN: 978-1-925999-99-0   ebook

Designer: PublishMyBookOnline
A catalogue record for this book is available from the
National Library of Australia.

Also available as an ebook from major ebook vendors.

Table of Contents

INTRODUCTION

Learning from the Past

E ver since COVID-19 was declared a pandemic on 11 March 2020, the world has been thrown into chaos and confusion. Lockdowns were mandated and citizens sheltered at home. Businesses were closed, shops shuttered and city streets became eerily quiet. Unemployment rose, along with mental health impacts, as the economy collapsed and descended into recession. Stress, fear and anxiety have swept the world like a wildfire, robbing people of a joyful life.

But have we been told the whole truth about this disease, or just a one-sided view? This book uncovers hidden truths that help people reclaim peace of mind, freedom of spirit and sovereignty over their lives.

The story begins in March 2020, highlighting the intense fear this disease has generated. It concludes with what has been learnt from previous pandemics and what people can learn from COVID-19, especially in the area of healthcare and technology. There are three parts to this book: Part One: The problem—killer pandemic and how it evolved. Part Two: The reaction—treatments and strategies. Part Three: The solution—building hope and resilience.

I have included a short story of my lived experience during the pandemic at the start of each chapter.

At the beginning of the pandemic, it was predicted that people would be dying like flies with the remainder living in fear of being infected or infecting others. Fear triggers a paralysis in rational thinking and citizens surrendered to the dictates of authoritarian institutions and governments, believing that science and those in positions of power know best. Time has proven that fear of the disease itself is largely unfounded because much of what we've been told by medical and political authorities is not grounded in good science.

The mathematical modelling that informed political and medical decisions in the highest levels of governments and bureaucracy was grossly overestimated, said Ivor Cummins in his YouTube video.[1] The lethality of COVID-19 was based on modelling that was, 'Catastrophically high in its estimations. It was out by a factor of 15+ and that's what threw the world into turmoil,' he said.

Aside from this initial travesty, there have been fundamental flaws in data acquisition, leading to an artificially high number of COVID-19 cases, such as those 'assumed' to have the disease included in the case numbers. There have also been breaches in the rules of infectiology and reporting, such as the many deaths being reported as COVID-19 fatalities irrespective of what the patient died from.[2] From around October 2020, the Centers for Disease Control and Prevention (CDC) combined COVID-19 deaths with pneumonia and flu under a new category: PIC (pneumonia, influenza and COVID),[3] making it difficult to determine the accurate number of deaths due to COVID-19 alone.

4

There are, however, other concerns, such as the British government's Medicines and Healthcare Products Regulatory Agency (MHRA) finding it necessary to utilise Artificial Intelligence (AI) software to keep track of everyone who is killed or injured after a future massive COVID-19 vaccine rollout. If potential COVID-19 vaccines are safe and up to 95% effective, as suggested by some current clinical trials, why is the MHRA describing this AI acquisition as one of 'extreme urgency' in its tender, explaining, '… if the MHRA does not implement the AI tool, it will be unable to process these ADRs [Adverse Drug Reactions] effectively. This will hinder its ability to rapidly identify potential safety issues with the COVID-19 vaccine and represents a direct threat to patient life and public health.'[4] Does the British government know something that the people haven't been told? Or are they withholding information because they're fearful that such disclosure may reduce the compliance of vaccine uptake by the general public?

Fear has been used as a weapon to control people—to manipulate and force them to succumb to an economic system in which personal and world affairs are dictated by technocrats. These ultra-wealthy elites, scientists and technicians aim to dominate the global population and the allocation of resources through the use of technology such as AI and big data analytics. Embedded in this system is the suppression of science by the medical-political complex for financial and political gain. Corruption is rampant. The pandemic emergency has shown how easily this network of corporations can be manipulated, aggrandising and enriching those in power. Politicians and industry, including scientists and health experts, are responsible for 'opportunistic embezzlement', and human life is expendable.

Robert F. Kennedy, Jr. Chair of the Children's Health Defense, said at a press conference in Berlin on 28 August 2020, 'For many years totalitarian or authoritarian states have used the power of fear to engineer compliance in populations ... All the rulers need to do is to tell the people that there's something they need to be fearful of. Point a finger at that source of their fear and you can make human beings do anything you want. You can make them go to the slaughter like sheep; you can make them obey.'[5]

Totalitarianism is on the rise and marching forward at an alarming rate. Is the fair go, fair share and fair say of democracy doomed? Australia's Foreign Minister, Marise Payne, said, '... it was troubling that some countries were "using the pandemic to undermine liberal democracy and promote their own, more authoritarian models,"'[6] and she specifically targeted China and Russia for spreading disinformation, which leads to confusion and fear.

Humanity has reached a crossroad—turn left for the Great Reset to bring about global communism and the complete enslavement of the human race worldwide, or turn right for the Great Awakening—a pro-liberty crusade rising rapidly to counter socio-political corruption and the suppression of science. People need to choose whether they will embrace the dictatorship of communism or the liberty of democracy.

The term 'fear appeal' is used in psychology, sociology and marketing to motivate people to take a prescribed action, endorse a particular policy or buy a certain product. Research has been undertaken in public health on how to frighten people to 'do the right thing' and get vaccinated against COVID-19. It's based on the premise that to successfully implement global vaccinations you must highlight the threat and keep it uppermost in people's minds. COVID-19 provided that threat.

This threat must also be made personal for maximum effect and has been achieved by enforcing lockdowns, the wearing of masks, closing businesses and keeping children home from school. Potential future directives that all people must be vaccinated and digitally tracked before they can travel overseas or even resume a normal life at home adds further to the 'fear appeal'.

Fear causes confusion and anxiety and, on reaching a certain point, depression sets in, according to Dr Peter Breggin, and people will do just about anything to get relief.[7]

The great scientist, Albert Einstein, is quoted as saying, 'Everything is energy. Your thought begins it, your emotion amplifies it and your action increases the momentum.' This is how our thoughts create our reality. This is how fear has been used as a weapon. Create the problem, the reaction is predictable and the solution is in their favour!

We can disempower the energy of fear by refusing to subscribe to it. A hot-air balloon (dominating entity) needs hot-air energy (fear) to keep it afloat. When we remove the hot air, the balloon comes crashing down. We can change our circumstances by changing our thoughts and, when we do so, we can change our lives.

The biggest influences in our reality have been news programs with a culture of left-wing bias and similarly slanted social media platforms with the proliferation of often misleading and conflicting information. This is part of the disinformation campaign Marise Payne was referring to, as previously discussed. This doesn't have to be our reality. We can 'disconnect' ourselves from this influence by not paying attention to it and instead, tune into information or listen to music that resonates best with us and our individual thoughts.

In writing this manuscript, I am indebted to Wayne Dyer's teachings in his book *Change Your Thoughts—Change Your Life: Living the Wisdom of the Tao.* His theoretical and practical applications of the *Tao Te Ching* are food for contemplative thought and a balm for jagged nerves. Do you feel overwhelmed by everything that is happening in our world at this particular time? Do you feel fearful of the future and what it may bring? Are you being confronted with conflicting information daily and don't know what to believe? If so, it's completely understandable, but there's hope for a better future if we learn to trust our intuition and do what's right for us.

Firstly, we need to ask ourselves, 'Is what I am being told by conventional wisdom in my best interests as a patient/citizen, or is the information being heavily promoted more beneficial for someone or something else? Is there another agenda?' Many highly-credentialed experts in both traditional and natural medicine offer a different perspective from the mainstream narrative. They should be getting a hearing too, but they aren't because there's too much demonising and censorship from the other side. By uncovering hidden truths and learning to tap into our own innate wisdom, we can move forward in our lives with courage and confidence.

Secondly, for peace to prevail in our troubled world, it's important to balance our understanding of both sides of the COVID story—the yin and the yang. We are being bombarded daily by fearful paternalistic messages of yang—case numbers are rising, but we never hear anything about the yin, the feminine side—the death rates are falling, despite rubbery statistics and exaggerated daily tolls.[8] Both these facts are true—they are two sides of the same story. We just need to listen to both sides of the story, be conscious of the feelings we perceive and what resonates with us as our truth and work quietly with that.

The classification of a COVID-19 death has become more elastic over time, as have the rules of infectiology and reporting, and governments of different nations are adopting their own mandates. WHO stipulates that a COVID death is someone who died of the disease, or is 'assumed' to have died of it, or where COVID may have 'contributed' to the death, even if that person died of another cause.[9] In the UK and elsewhere, COVID-19 is listed as the cause of death if a patient was diagnosed with the disease, fully recovered, and died of something unrelated within 28 days afterwards because COVID-19 may have 'contributed' to their death.[10] Prior to August 2020, the government in England had been reporting all deaths after a positive test as a coronavirus death, irrespective of what the patient died from.

People who die with COVID-19 and people who die from COVID-19 are lumped in the one statistic [11] together with all 'assumed' cases and all those who died of other causes, such as cancer, where lack of access to treatment caused by the pandemic may have contributed to their death. In England and other countries, COVID-19 'survivors are never considered truly recovered from the disease'.[12] The authors of this article further state, 'Health Secretary

Matt Hancock has ordered Public Health England to review the way it counts deaths because of a 'statistical flaw' that meant officials were 'over-exaggerating' the daily toll.' The rules around transparency, infectiology and reporting need to change to reflect genuine COVID-19 deaths—people dying from medically-diagnosed COVID-19 only, and these need to be adopted by all nations worldwide to understand the true impact of the virus and the responses necessary to counteract it rather than relying on political propaganda for an inflated best-case scenario.

As more people learn to tap into their innate wisdom, the less we will be led astray by political propaganda. We will learn to trust our gut instincts and know what is right for us rather than being told what's best for us. We will learn to be masters of our destiny, doing what's best in the spirit of goodwill rather than being led passively like lambs to the slaughter. We will intuitively know what others are thinking and if we're being told the truth. Things aren't always what they seem—they are what we perceive. Our perception is our reality and our reality is what we believe.

My background in social welfare and nutrition, working for people with disabilities, has taught me to look for the disease, the feeling of uneasiness behind the disease, when offering holistic solutions in any given situation. Fear is a disease behind the COVID-19 pandemic, and disease creates unintended consequences, such as mental health impacts. When we recognise the nature of thoughts as energy, we understand that fear is being used as a weapon and it can be neutralised by learning to be resilient and no longer subscribing to it. By changing fearful thoughts to something pleasant, such as writing a daily gratitude list, being grateful for what we DO have in life, the energy frequency of the space-time continuum changes, and miracles happen.

Taoist philosophy teaches us to be like water, 'Instead of resisting problems and adversity, try letting things be. Be like water and find ways to flow around obstacles with ease and grace.' When water in a rock pool is calm and settled, the pebbles at the bottom can be seen clearly. If it's stirred and agitated, the water becomes cloudy and vision is impaired. The same is true of life—we can achieve what we desire, but we don't have to stir the pot to get it. Focus and intention are much more important—where focus goes, energy flows. Tony Robbins, motivational speaker and author of several books including *Awaken the Giant Within*, is a firm believer in focusing on what we really want in life with a clear goal in mind and purpose and meaning behind it. 'When you learn to focus your energy, amazing things happen,'[13] he said.

This book is ideally suited to people who embrace a wellness model of healthcare; those who like to think independently and put faith in their own judgement. Readers are provided with information that uncovers hidden truths highlighting different perspectives of the evolving pandemic. By offering such information, readers will be given choices. They will be empowered to make informed decisions regarding their own lives and the environment in which they live, giving them the freedom to journey forward in whatever direction they choose.

I love the way Albert Einstein thinks, and one of my favourite quotes of his is, 'Education is not the learning of facts, but the training of the mind to think.' I hope the information in this book will, at least, provide you with something to think about. It may just change our world and save your life.

PART 1

The Problem: Killer Pandemic and how it Evolved

CHAPTER 1

The Sneaky Thief

It was the best of times, it was the worst of times

There was something in the air

I t came out of nowhere, like a thief in the night, catching us all unaware. The first inkling I had that COVID-19 was not just someone else's news was when I flew into Sydney from rural New South Wales on 7 March 2020, about to embark on a rail holiday in beautiful New Zealand. It was Saturday and the streets were eerily quiet; so unusual. Normally city life is hustle and bustle, even on weekends, but this quietness had an ominous feel to it. It seemed that something wasn't quite right.

Before flying out for my much-anticipated New Zealand holiday, I went to a major shopping centre at Chatswood to do some last-minute shopping. Typically, this multicultural suburb, populated predominantly with people of Asian descent, is jam-packed with business personnel and consumers during weekdays and on weekends. But not on this occasion; shoppers were few and far between—no queues, no foreign languages, no buskers and seemingly no life.

What's going on? I wondered. It seemed like I had stepped into a parallel universe and what was familiar was suddenly now very strange indeed. I tried not to think about it too much; I didn't want to spoil my holiday with negative thoughts so I purchased my items and made my way back to the hotel where I was staying overnight.

The next morning was Sunday, the day of my departure. Because it was raining, I decided to get a taxi to the airport as I didn't want to battle with crowded trains in the wet. There was little traffic on the road and hardly a soul to be seen anywhere. It was a breeze run to the airport. I was starting to think that the rumbling of coronavirus in the distance was more serious than I had been told. *Perhaps martial law was in place and someone had forgotten to tell me about it.*

I checked in for my flight to Auckland. I noticed the staff were not exactly friendly, and service seemed to be a chore. But in hindsight, they may have had other things on their minds. Perhaps they'd been told they would not have a job soon because of coronavirus.

Despite this niggling doubt, I was excited. I had never been to New Zealand before and my rail tour through picture-postcard landscapes promised to be quite an adventure. I did wonder, however, just how adventurous my holiday would become.

The Australian Government was alerted about the new viral outbreak in China at the beginning of the year but didn't pay much attention to it until the World Health Organisation declared a pandemic on 11 March 2020. By this time, I was 'across the ditch' in another country, meeting people from all walks of life and having a wonderful time in the land of the long white cloud. Despite a heightened awareness of the seriousness of this disease, I was not going to let fear spoil my long-awaited holiday. I was determined to live life to the fullest come what may and deal with any hiccups if and when they arose. The main issue, as it happened, was the cancellation of my return ticket from Christchurch to Sydney and having to reschedule my flight via Auckland to Sydney due to the implementation of the New Zealand lockdown.

What is COVID-19 and what are the symptoms?

COVID-19 is the disease caused by the novel coronavirus SARS-CoV-2, which is Severe Acute Respiratory Syndrome (SARS), Coronavirus (CoV) type 2. 'CO' stands for corona, 'V' for virus, 'ID' for infectious disease, and '-19' refers to the year that this disease was first reported. It's a highly infectious respiratory illness that, we are told, has not appeared previously in our world population. SARS-CoV-2 belongs to a large family of coronaviruses that cause illnesses ranging from the common cold to more severe diseases such as SARS and MERS.

Infection with this coronavirus can cause symptoms ranging anywhere from mild to severe. It affects people in different ways, with the most common symptoms being a fever, dry cough and tiredness. Less common symptoms include aches and pains, sore throat, headache and the loss of taste or smell. More serious symptoms include difficulty breathing and shortness of breath, chest pain or feeling of pressure in the chest and loss of speech or movement.

According to the World Health Organisation (WHO), older adults and people with existing health conditions are more likely to be at higher risk for severe complications, which can be life-threatening.

Where did it come from, when and how?

The first known case of COVID-19 was reported in December 2019, emerging from Wuhan, China, and has been genetically identified as being 96% horseshoe bat coronavirus.[14]

It was initially declared and is still maintained by some, that this virus is zoonotic in origin, a disease that's transmitted between species from animals to humans, and this occurred via the wet markets in Wuhan. Others claim that this virus is of animal origin, specifically bats, but was assisted in a laboratory to obtain increased adaptability and transmissibility by tampering with the genome and leaked from a biosecurity laboratory in Wuhan, China.

The Chinese government, its affiliates and supporters, maintain that SARS-CoV-2 occurred due to natural evolution. SARS-CoV-1 was identified 17 years ago in the Guangdong province of southern China. Natural evolution such as this, according to Dr Judy Mikovits, PhD, a highly trained virologist with 40 years of research experience, normally takes approximately 800 years.

If this virus did originate from the wet market in Wuhan and naturally evolved, jumping from animals to humans at lightning speed, then we can deal with this catastrophe by shutting down all wet markets worldwide. If, on the other hand, this virus emerged from animal origin via tampering in a laboratory, as some say, then we have a lot more to be concerned about; our future may be very bleak indeed.

Pandemic declared

Authorities in China first informed WHO of the Wuhan virus on 31 December 2019. The director-general of WHO, Tedros Adhanom Ghebreyesus, declared SARS-CoV-2 to be a Public Health Emergency of International Concern on 30 January 2020, but this was not taken seriously until 11 March 2020 when a pandemic was declared. SARS and MERS are also zoonotic coronaviruses, but unlike SARS-CoV-2, did not have pandemic potential.

When a pandemic was declared by WHO, countries were ordered into lockdown, businesses ground to a halt, people isolated at home and, by this time, thousands of individuals had died. Panic hit our shores. We were not allowed out of our homes for anything other than purchasing food, exercise, caring for the sick or if we were working for what was considered an essential service. A social distance of one and a half metres was required to be kept between all people at all times and signs were placed on the floor at supermarket checkouts and other stores to keep shoppers separated. Mandated orders were issued, social gatherings were banned and restrictions were placed on the distance people could travel from their own community, which were policed, and fines were issued for breaches.

We had everything before us until COVID-19 landed on our doorstep, along with the dire consequences it imposed. Statistical modelling predicted that millions of people worldwide would die in a catastrophe similar to that of the Spanish Flu in 1918–1919. The initial medical advice based on modelling at the beginning of the pandemic, given for example by Neil Ferguson of the Imperial College, London, projected 500,000 deaths for Britain.[15] This prompted

British Prime Minister Boris Johnson to immediately lock down his people and the economy. People worldwide became fearful and submitted themselves to mandatory lockdowns, social distancing and testing, generally with high obedience. As time moved on, compliance has waned and more people are flouting the rules. They are getting tired of the restrictive lockdowns, frustrated with the escalating unemployment, and mental health issues are of grave concern, as we will see in later chapters.

The origins of the PCR test and its application

The reverse transcription polymerase chain reaction (RT-PCR) test has been used as the 'gold standard' to detect SARS-CoV-2 in the population worldwide and diagnose COVID-19, even though this test was never designed for this purpose. Dr Kary Mullis (1944–2019), who shared the Nobel Peace Prize for Chemistry in 1993 for his invention of the PCR test, didn't recommend it for the diagnosis of infection.[16] It can't distinguish between inactive viruses and live, reproductive ones.[17] The purpose of this technology is for research—to replicate DNA sequences and not test for coronavirus infections.

> 'An in-depth investigation reveals clear scientific evidence proving that these tests are not accurate and create a statistically significant percentage of false positives. **Positive results more likely indicate "ordinary respiratory diseases like the common cold."**'[18]

The Australian government has admitted that this test is flawed but the best we have.[19] Legal proceedings in Lisbon, Portugal, ruled on 11 November 2020 that the PCR test was not fit for purpose[20] and, despite being heavily promoted by Professor Christian Drosten, Head of the Institute for Virology, Berlin, and WHO, is 'not valid to detect coronavirus infection' and should not be used as a basis to mandate partial or nationwide lockdowns.[21] Dr Pascal Sacre, a critical care physician in Belgium and one of many thousands of angry doctors objecting to the PCR test being used to diagnose COVID-19, said:

> 'This misuse of RT-PCR technique is used as a **relentless and intentional strategy by some governments**, supported by scientific safety councils and by the dominant media, **to justify excessive measures** such as the violation of a large number of constitutional rights, the destruction of the economy with the bankruptcy of entire active sectors of society, the degradation of living conditions for a large number of ordinary citizens, under the pretext of a pandemic **based on a number of positive RT-PCR tests, and not on a real number of patients.**'[22]

How the PCR test was chosen

Professor Christian Drosten is also a member of the editorial board of *Eurosurveillance*, a premier European medical journal, and together with Victor M Corman and colleagues, published a study on 23 January 2020 claiming to have developed the first effective test for detecting SAR-CoV-2.[23] This study was submitted to *Eurosurveillance* for publication on 21 January 2020, accepted on 22 January 2020 and available online on 23 January 2020. This paper states that no conflicts of interest were declared. It is highly unlikely that a peer review could have taken place in this short timeframe, and surprisingly, this test was adopted and recommended by WHO on 17 January 2020 before the paper was even published.[24]

At the crux of the PCR problem is the arbitrary cycling process where nucleotides, tiny fragments of DNA or RNA, are replicated until there is something large enough to identify. This replication is carried out in cycles with each cycle doubling the amount of genetic material. The cycle threshold, or Ct value, is the number of cycles the test passes through until something can be identified.[25] The higher the Ct value, the less reliable the results. There has been no benchmark set for a standard operating protocol to determine whether a test is positive or negative based on the Ct value used to identify infection.

Pieter Borger, PhD, is an expert in the molecular biology of gene expression and has worked for several research institutes worldwide. He and 21 other highly-respected research scientists published a call for *Eurosurveillance* to retract the January 23, 2020 Corman-Drosten paper highlighting 10 major flaws in relation to the research, some of which include:

'The test cannot discriminate between the whole virus and viral fragments … The PCR products have not been validated at the molecular level … The PCR test contains neither a unique positive control to evaluate its specificity for SARS-CoV-2 nor a negative control to exclude the presence of other coronaviruses … The test design in the Corman-Drosten paper is so vague and flawed that one can go in dozens of different directions; nothing is standardized and there is no SOP … We find severe conflicts of interests for at least four authors, in addition to the fact that two of the authors of the Corman-Drosten paper (Christian Drosten and Chantal Reusken) are members of the editorial board of Eurosurveillance …'[26]

This damning report further states:

'These types of virological diagnostic tests must be based on a SOP [Standard Operational Protocol], including a validated and fixed number of PCR cycles (Ct value) after which a sample is deemed positive or negative. The maximum reasonably reliable Ct value is 30 cycles. Above a Ct of 35 cycles, rapidly increasing numbers of false positives must be expected.'

A study conducted by Jaafar et al. found that when running PCR tests with 35 cycles or more, the accuracy dropped to three percent, meaning that up to 97% of positive COVID-19 results could be false positives.[27] Yet WHO and Drosten recommend a Ct of 45 cycles[28] and the FDA and CDC recommend running the PCR test at a Ct of 40.[29] Dr Anthony Fauci, director of the National Institutes of Allergy and Infectious Diseases (NAID) admitted in a Twitter video that a Ct value over 35 is going to be detecting dead nucleotides and not a living virus.[30] Is it really much wonder that COVID-19 cases are increasing worldwide when such high Ct values are used and there is no universal Standard Operational Protocol to guide the testing procedure?

WHO finally admitted on 14 December 2020 that there is a 'problem' with the PCR test. It has a 'hit and miss process with way too many false positives'. This admission 'comes in the wake of international lawsuits exposing the incompetence and malfeasance of public health officials and policy makers for reliance on a diagnostic test *not fit for purpose*',[31] resulting in worldwide lockdowns, economic devastation and human suffering of enormous magnitude. WHO has known of this testing irregularity for some time but only reported it in December 2020. Could the reason be that a vaccine has recently become available and WHO can now change the guidelines stipulating that PCR tests be run at 25–30 cycles instead of the more commonly 35+, in which case, 'positive cases' will plummet, justifying how well the vaccine is working?

The PCR test is a tool that can be easily manipulated, as confirmed by the inventor Dr Kary Mullis when he said, 'with PCR, if you do it well, you can find almost anything in anybody.'[32]

The Ct value of an individual's test result is available to patients if they ask for it, according to Dr Fauci in his Twitter video.[33]

Flattening the Gompertz curve

Ivor Cummins has an engineering degree from the University College Dublin, Ireland, and spent 25 years in corporate technical leadership and management, specialising in leading teams in complex problem-solving situations. A major health challenge forced him to direct his focus on health, where he uses engineering problem-solving rigour and scientific method to answer some of the more complex questions of everyday life.

In his YouTube video mentioned previously, 'Viral Issue Crucial Update Sept 8th: The Science, Logic and Data Explained', viewed over 1.5 million times, Ivor said you get a Gompertz curve in viral epidemics, where growth is slowest at the start and the end, with a big peak in the middle, and these curves are 'baked-in'. They happen all the time. 'Community immunity, the passing of the susceptible, the seasonal changes in the virome and other factors naturally dictate this curve,' he said.

When a virus first hits a community, it rapidly spreads to around 20% of the population. These people are those less immune, such as the susceptible elderly. The virus then stumbles over immune people, unable to gain traction, before it falls rapidly. This is when you get the turning of the curve, or the 'flattening', and this is entirely normal, he said, with coronaviruses and influenza.

There was a very 'soft' flu season in 2019, right up to early 2020, according to Ivor. 'We really had a lot of fragile elderly people who would have otherwise sadly passed.' When COVID struck, there was a lot of 'dry tinder'—a new term that is being used now—and all those aged, susceptible and comorbid people were around to be sadly hit with the coronavirus.

Lockdown was a massive mistake and a failure of science

'The lockdown effectively had no impact [on the death rate] even though the belief system is that it should. Sorry guys, the science is tough that way,' said Ivor Cummins in the abovementioned video. He said there are several published papers on lockdown analysis now and we're seeing more all the time, even in *The Wall Street Journal*, where scientists are slowly and reluctantly acknowledging that lockdown was a massive mistake and will cause more deaths than lives saved. It's the same with masks, Ivor went on to say. 'There has been no measurable impact between mandatory mask orders and no masks.'

Donald L Luskin wrote an opinion piece in the *Wall Street Journal*, highlighting how two large-scale experiments in public health, the first in March/April 2020, at the beginning of the pandemic, and the second, since April 2020, have proved that locking down people and the economy didn't contain the spread of the disease and re-opening it didn't unleash a second wave of infections. Donald Luskin states, 'It turns out that lockdowns correlated with a greater spread of the virus. States with longer, stricter lockdowns also had larger COVID outbreaks. The five places with the hardest lockdowns—the District of Columbia, New York, Michigan, New Jersey and Massachusetts—had the heaviest caseloads.'[34] Melbourne, Australia, would fall into this category too with its harsh lockdown instigated by a dictatorial premier and maintained by a full-flown police state and a night-time curfew.

It turns out, according to the abovementioned article, that the negative correlation remains, even when including other factors such as 'population density, age, ethnicity, prevalence of nursing homes, general health or temperature'. The only factor that seems to make a significant difference, the author said, is 'the intensity of mass-transit use', indicating large numbers of people in confined and enclosed spaces, such as on ships, in public transport and elevators in high-rise buildings and nursing homes. This is where problems lie for the spread of disease.

In a research paper published by *The Lancet*, the authors state, 'Rapid border closures, full lockdowns, and wide-spread testing were not associated with COVID-19 mortality per million people.'[35]

Simon Wood from the University of Edinburgh, UK, said in a research paper, 'The most notable feature of the results is that fatal infections are inferred to be in substantial decline before lockdown.'[36]

The authors of a preprint research article have highlighted, 'Stay at home orders, closure of all non-[essential] businesses and requiring the wearing of facemasks or coverings in public was not associated with any independent additional impact. Our results could help inform strategies for coming out of lockdown.'[37]

Lockdown compromises individual and community immunity

An Oxford epidemiologist, Professor Sunetra Gupta, warned in June 2020 that extended lockdowns could damage the human immune system and leave people more vulnerable to disease. In a *Daily Mail* Australia article Professor Gupta said, 'Intense social distancing could leave people unexposed to germs and not develop defences against new viruses.' She used the analogy, 'If we return to the point where we have no exposure, society would be like clumps of trees waiting to be set ablaze.' She went on to say, 'The kind of immunity that protects you against very severe symptoms and death can be acquired by exposure to related pathogens rather than the virus itself.'[38]

Lockdowns can have a negative effect, Ivor Cummins said in his previously mentioned video, 'Viral Issue Crucial Update Sept 8th: The Science, Logic and Data Explained'. 'They're going to cause way more cancer deaths from late diagnoses, way more malnourishment and suicide and dreadful impacts due to destroying economies. They are taking away our cherished freedoms and causing terrible societal impacts.' This is reinforced by Professor Ian Hickie, co-director of the Brain and Mind Centre at the University of Sydney who said, 'The predicted increase of suicides is 25 per cent each year for the next five years. ... It's an enormous number. It will be a massively bigger death toll than COVID.'[39] These and other issues will be discussed further in chapter five.

But these are not the only detriments. For the first time in history, healthy people have been isolated, and in some cases for extended periods, such as in Melbourne, Australia, and other countries that have had hard lockdowns. Normally in summer, viruses circulate with very low mortality, allowing people to build immunity and, according to Ivor Cummins, that helps to protect the elderly and frail during the following winter, traditionally the flu season. Stopping this natural immune-boosting capacity during the summer months by keeping people in lockdown has the potential to make the next 'wave' during the following winter much worse than it needs to be in terms of death and injury of the susceptible and the weak, the very ones we want to protect, commented Ivor Cummins in his video. 'So, wouldn't it be ironic if what actually would have been a mid-range winter actually became worse because we have not developed the normal ancestral evolutionary summer period community immunity. Now that would be an enormous backfire,' he said.

Even WHO is now discouraging lockdowns, Dr David Nabarro, WHO's special envoy on COVID-19, said in an *ABC News* article, 'We really do appeal to all world leaders: stop using lockdown as your primary control method. We in the World Health Organisation do not advocate lockdowns as the primary means of control of this virus. The only time we believe a lockdown is justified is to buy time to reorganise, regroup, rebalance your resources, protect your health workers who are exhausted, but by and large, we'd rather not do it.'[40]

The WHO recommends self-responsibility—engaging people and trusting them to do the right thing rather than using coercion, if at all possible. These measures include 'physical distancing, proper face-masking, hand/cough/ surface hygiene, self-isolating when ill and shielding those most at risk.'[41]

Ivor Cummins said, 'Doing things that are not based on good science, such as lockdown, and continuing them all summer could have pretty terrible unforeseen consequences, in which case, the people pushing this would tend to have blood on their hands next winter.' Unintended consequences—damage, injury and death, happen when you don't follow good science.

Stockpiling food and other essentials

People scrambled to stockpile food and other items such as toilet paper in the early days of lockdown. Why toilet paper vanished remains a mystery; it became as scarce as hen's teeth. COVID-19 affects the respiratory system, not the gastrointestinal plumbing! Many of our popular food staples and necessities were purchased en masse from major centres and small regional towns, depleting local supplies, and shipped to China and other countries.

What is going on, and why? Is it because the People's Republic of China and its political alliances have a serious shortage or was the created scarcity aimed at us to undermine our confidence and comfort? By destabilising a country to make it weaker, the oppressor's attack will be stronger. It's an old tactic that was used in previous wars. The supply chain, including food delivery to the enemy, was severed, making them too weak to fight, and overcoming resistance became easy.

Lizzie Collingham, historian, said the following about World War II (WWII), 'The war was not about the triumph of democracy over fascism. It was the victory of adequate diet over starvation.'[42] Japanese soldiers attempted to seize Papua New Guinea in their advance along the Kokoda Track during WWII but were forced to retreat—hungry, ill and weary due to their food supply lines being disrupted. 'On the overland retreat from Sio to Wewak, tens of thousands of Japanese soldiers perished, mostly as a result of sickness and malnutrition.'[43]

Statistics and demographics

Data from several global studies, including the Centres for Disease Control and Prevention (CDC) suggest that 81% of COVID-19 positive people will have mild to moderate symptoms, 14% will have more severe symptoms and 5% of patients will be critically ill, requiring intensive care.[44] Elderly people in nursing homes and people of colour are at a higher risk of severe complications as a result of this disease and this may be due, in part, to a pre-existing vitamin D deficiency.[45] Vitamin D deficiency in the elderly and people of colour will be discussed further in chapter four—alternative treatment.

In an article published in *The Lancet* on 30 March 2020, researchers collected individual case data from patients who died from COVID-19 in China and concluded that the infection fatality rate for COVID-19, while minimal for healthy young people, escalates with age. This study identified cohorts 50 to 59, 60 to 69, 70 to 79, and above 80 years of age, with estimated infection fatality rates of 0.6%, 1.9%, 4.3%, and 7.8% respectively.[46] Multiple disorders are often prevalent in an ageing population and some young people have pre-existing conditions, such as obesity and diabetes, and the complication of these comorbidities increases the death rate.

An Australian Department of Health paper reported, 'Comorbidities were common in those COVID-19 cases admitted to Australian sentinel hospitals (general ward or ICU), with 78% recording at least one of the specified comorbidities; only 9% recorded no comorbidity. The proportion of hospitalised cases with no known comorbidity recorded in U.S. hospital surveillance system COVID-NET was also reportedly 9%.'[47] This indicates that the healthier people are, the less likely they are to succumb to COVID-19 or be severely affected by it. Most of these comorbidities are lifestyle diseases which can be either prevented or reversed by paying attention to diet and lifestyle factors. The importance of lifestyle factors such as diet, nutrition, exercise, rest and relaxation in building immunity—our natural defence system against any disease—is discussed in chapter four.

In Australia, as of 03 February 2021, 909 lives have been lost, mostly in Victoria, due to COVID-19 and, unfortunate as it is, most of those have been elderly people with pre-existing comorbidities. But the absolute seriousness of this disease, the infection fatality rate (relatively low) compared with the total number of cases (proportionately much higher), is getting a little questionable when compared with the mental health impacts that COVID-19 has caused. Many people are identified in total cases with COVID-19, and many people die with COVID-19, but not from it. The tragedy is, people who die with COVID-19 are still recorded as a COVID-19 death, even if their primary cause of death was heart disease or cancer, for example, and this skews the figures.

If someone dies in a motor vehicle accident and they were subsequently diagnosed with COVID-19, the cause of death on their death certificate will be recorded as COVID-19. This is a WHO directive. '**COVID-19** should be recorded on the medical certificate of cause of death for ALL decedents where the disease caused, or is assumed to have caused, or contributed to death.'[48] This subjective nature of recording COVID-19 deaths is the very 'liberal approach' the White House Coronavirus Task Force is taking, according to Dr Deborah Birx, Coronavirus Response Coordinator.[49]

Dr Anthony Fauci, once a prominent member of the White House Coronavirus Task Force, and director of the National Institute of Allergy and Infectious Diseases (NAID), admitted, 'The overall clinical consequences of COVID-19 may ultimately be more akin to those of a severe seasonal influenza, which has a case fatality rate of approximately 0.1%.'[50] WHO director-general, Dr Tedros Adhanom Ghebreyesus, has reinforced this finding by saying at a news conference in Geneva, 'It appears that COVID-19 is not as deadly as other coronaviruses, including SARS and MERS,' adding that 'more than 80% of patients have mild disease and will recover'.[51]

In the initial stages of this disease, not enough was known as far as reliable case studies were concerned. The goalposts kept moving depending on who you spoke to regarding the actual death rate of this disease and the long-term medical consequences. 'The big caveat here is that researchers are trying to hit a moving target and could be missing by a mile. The actual lethality of this disease will become clearer in the next few weeks as more data, especially from population screening with antibody tests, comes in.'[52]

Data is now available and COVID-19 has had no additional effect on the overall number of deaths. It's the goals that have moved. Genevieve Briand is an Assistant Director at Johns Hopkins University in Applied Economics. She has analysed data from the US CDC regarding the percentages of total deaths in the US per age group from mid-March to mid-September 2020 and her findings reveal there has been no increase in the number of overall deaths in the US during this period. Deaths from chronic diseases such as cancer, heart attack and stroke have been re-classified as COVID-19 deaths reducing the number of deaths in the chronic disease cohort. The increase in deaths classified as COVID-19 fatalities has increased in a corresponding manner making the total number of deaths from all causes about the same as before the pandemic. 'Therefore, according to Briand, not only has COVID-19 had no effect on the percentage of deaths of older people, but it has also not increased the total number of deaths.'[53]

The flu has practically disappeared off the radar globally during 2020 season, while COVID-19 cases have soared. Social distancing and improved hygiene may have helped but Stephen Lendman, research analyst and author, believes 'Covid is "seasonal influenza" in disguise — in the US and worldwide.'[54] 'Mask wearing,' he said, 'is ineffective and potentially harmful to health … Aerosol spores are minuscule. Able to penetrate all masks and [the] concentrate beneath them risks greater harm to wearers than avoiding their use.' More on masks later in this chapter.

A study was conducted in Japan on 376 people six months after they had recovered from COVID-19 and it was discovered from blood samples that they had developed immunity to the disease. Seventy-one percent of these participants described their symptoms as mild, 19% had moderate symptoms, 6% had severe symptoms and 4% showed no symptoms at all. A follow-up study will be conducted 12 months after these participants had been infected to see if they still have antibodies to the disease.[55]

The Infection Fatality Rate (IFR), discussed in more detail below, is the most crucial metric in determining the mortality of COVID-19 and this varies according to age. A study was conducted to determine the IFR across all age groups to inform public health policies and communications to help protect vulnerable groups. The results of this study indicate the IFR for different age groups as follows:

Children 10 years and under—0.002%
Young adults 25 years and under—0.01%
Adults 55 years—0.04%
Adults 65 years—1.4%
Adults 75 years—4.6%
Adults 85 years—15%

This study highlighted, '… the overall IFR for COVID-19 should not be viewed as a fixed parameter, but as intrinsically linked to the age-specific pattern of infections. Consequently, public health measures to mitigate infections in older adults could substantially decrease total deaths'.[56] This also means that it's intrinsically linked to the state of health of the individual and how well their immune system is working for them.

Average age of death from COVID-19 and all other causes is similar

Data analysed by experts at the Centre for Evidence-Based Medicine (CEBM) has revealed that the average age of deaths from COVID-19 is 82.4 years. 'The average age of those who have died from coronavirus in England and Wales since the start of the pandemic is 82.4 years old. Using data from the Office for National Statistics (ONS), researchers at the University of Oxford found that the median age of a COVID-19 fatality was slightly higher than the median age of those who died of other causes over the same period, which was 81.5.'[57]

The types of tests used

There are two main types of tests used to detect COVID-19 and they are the nucleic acid reverse transcriptase polymerase chain reaction (RT-PCR) test, which can potentially detect an active SARS-CoV-2 infection, and the COVID-19 serology test, which detects antibodies to this virus in the blood of the patient. The PCR test is obtained by a swab sample taken from the back of the nose and throat of the patient. The antibody test is obtained by the collection of a blood sample. According to the CDC, an antibody test may not show if you have a current infection because it can take from one to three weeks after infection for the human body to make antibodies.

How the total number of cases is calculated

There is confusion surrounding the authenticity and legitimacy of the COVID-19 tests, not only with the high rate of false positives and false negatives but also in how the public is being informed of the total number of cases.

COVID-19 diagnostic (PCR) and antibody tests are being combined in total cases, even when the two tests reveal different information and are used for different reasons.[58] The total number of cases is the combination of PCR and antibody tests, together with 'probable cases' that don't have a confirmed diagnosis but meet some criteria. A clearer explanation is as follows:

PCR test: The reverse transcriptase PCR tests are widely used to diagnose COVID-19 and to detect SARS-CoV-2 nucleic acid (RNA). A positive result is classed as a positive COVID-19 case, even if it's a false positive.

Antibody test: 'A positive [antibody] test result shows you may have antibodies from an infection with the virus that causes COVID-19. However, there is a chance a positive result means that you have antibodies from an infection with a virus from the same family of viruses (called coronaviruses)'[59] such as the one that causes the common cold. A positive antibody result is classed as a positive COVID-19 case, even though the antibodies may be from a previous common cold coronavirus!

Probable cases: Cases that meet some criteria such as patients having a 'sore throat and a headache' or 'cough' with either presumptive or no confirmatory laboratory evidence.[60] Probable cases are those 'assumed' to have the disease.

Total cases: The combination of diagnostic and antibody tests plus the number of 'probable' cases, and this is what is reported in the media.

Combining these three 'tests' conflates the numbers, compromising crucial metrics that politicians and health authorities depend on to reopen their economies. Until there is some uniform standard for testing criteria, it will be difficult to obtain accurate and reliable data.

The emperor has no clothes

Dr Malcolm Kendrick, a Scottish doctor and author said, 'It seems that Dr Fauci just got mixed up with the terminology [in relation to COVID-19] ... Dr Fauci, the CDC, his co-authors, the National Institute of Allergy and Infectious Diseases, and the National Institutes of Health *and* the New England Journal of Medicine got case fatality rate and infection fatality rate mixed up with influenza. ... The truth is that this particular Emperor has no clothes on.'[61]

There is a huge difference between the **case** fatality rate and the **infection** fatality rate; a difference of a factor of 10, according to the numbers that have been modelled. When mathematical modellers were trying to determine the impact of COVID-19, 'They used a figure of approximately one percent as the *infection* rate. Not the case fatality rate. In doing so, they overestimated the likely impact of COVID by, at the very least, ten-fold,' Dr Kendrick said in the report referred to above.

Dr Anthony Fauci admitted in an editorial article in the *New England Journal of Medicine* referred to previously, 'COVID-19–Navigating the Uncharted', 'If one assumes that the number of asymptomatic or minimally symptomatic cases is several times as high as the number of reported cases, the case fatality rate may be considerably less than 1%. This suggests that the overall clinical consequences of Covid-19 may ultimately be more akin to those of a severe seasonal influenza (which has a case fatality rate of approximately 0.1%),' as mentioned previously.

Case fatality rate (CFR) is the ratio of the number of deaths divided by the number of confirmed (preferably by nucleic acid testing) *cases* of disease.[62] It's the proportion of deaths from a certain disease compared with the total number of people diagnosed with the disease. This means that anyone who died either with or from COVID-19 is included in the case fatality rate. The only figure that should be used for the case fatality rate is the people actually diagnosed with COVID-19 infection 'by nucleic acid testing' such as the PCR test which may or may not be accurate. The antibody tests are notoriously inaccurate and 'assumed' or 'contributed' cases have not been confirmed by medical diagnosis.

Infection fatality rate (IFR) 'Is the radio of deaths divided by the number of actual *infections* with SARS-CoV-2. Dr Kendrick says in his report referred to previously, 'The infection fatality rate is *the* measure of how many people who are infected [even those without symptoms, or very mild symptoms] who then die. **This is *the* crucial figure to know because it gives you an accurate assessment of the total number of deaths you are likely to see** [emphasis added].'

In the words of Dr Malcolm Kendrick in 'COVID—why terminology really, really matters':

'You want to know where Imperial College London really got their 1% infection fatality rate figure from? It seems clear that they got it from Anthony S Fauci and the *New England Journal of Medicine*, the highest impact journal in the world … Imperial College then used this wrong *NEJM* influenza case fatality rate 0.1%. It seems that they then compared this 0.1% figure to the reported COVID case fatality rate, estimated to be 1% and multiplied the impact of COVID by ten. ... So, we got Lockdown. The US used the Fauci figure and got locked down. The world used that figure and got locked down. **That figure just happens to be ten times too high** [emphasis added].'

Dr Kendrick points out that a catastrophic error has been made in the mathematical modelling of this disease and that it's nowhere near as deadly as we are being told. We're constantly hearing about the rising number of cases as more and more tests are being conducted, yet the number of proportionate deaths continues to fall. As Dr Kendrick said, 'I know it is going to be virtually impossible to walk the world back from having made such a ridiculous, stupid mistake. There are so many reputations at stake. The entire egg production of the world will be required to supply enough yolk to cover appropriate faces.'

Patients testing positive, negative or suspected

When patients test positive for COVID-19, they are required to self-isolate in their home or accommodation until public health officers advise that it's safe to return to normal activities. People testing negative are free to go about their normal activities, but if they've been in contact with someone testing positive to the disease, they are suspected of having contracted the disease and are required to self-isolate for 14 days or until public health authorities inform them that it's safe to return to normal activities.

'Tests, tests and more testing' is a mantra that we are hearing a lot about during this pandemic. We are told that social distancing measures also need to be accompanied by scaled-up testing capabilities and anyone with the slightest scratchy throat or hint of cough is strongly encouraged to get themselves tested. Drive-through and walk-through clinics have been set up in strategic locations across the nation such as in car parks and shopping centres. We are told that it is essential that we identify all cases of COVID-19 before we release the brakes on lockdowns and social restrictions.

On the flip side, coronavirus tests, mostly made in China, have exposed a huge lie where numbers are wildly exaggerated with false positives vastly outnumbering real positives and the official infection counts are being wildly overstated. The African nation of Tanzania sent samples to WHO for COVID-19 testing. Among the specimens that tested positive for this disease were samples from a goat, a papaya and a pheasant.[63] This seems incredible but, if believed, reveals the scientific fraud behind some coronavirus tests.

An Australian journalist with more than 30 years' experience working for leading publications said he tested positive for COVID-19, but that was not his main concern. This journalist, who chose to remain anonymous, said after multiple 'no caller ID' phone calls from the Department of Health, scamming, bungled tracing and a visit from the police, he believes this part of the COVID process is alarmingly flawed.[64]

Social disobedience and mass rallies

Indigenous people throughout Australia tacked onto the tailwind of COVID-19 to highlight their cause with outrage against police. They and their advocates were quick to seize the opportunity to raise awareness of their racial issues, particularly black deaths in custody, by organising mass rallies and protests over the June 2020 long weekend in major cities and some regional centres. The New South Wales Government tried to halt these proceedings in the interests of public health and safety. Premier Gladys Berejiklian took the matter to the Supreme Court, which initially ruled in favour of the NSW Government. However, an appeal saw this decision overturned and protesters were granted permission to conduct their rallies only 15 minutes before the long weekend protest marches were due to commence. It was a matter of social justice colliding with social restrictions, and the former won the day.

The NSW Government has expressed its dismay about social restrictions being flouted in mass protests and rallies, and the risk this poses for the broader community. Other politicians have urged protesters to seek avenues that don't compromise public health to get their message across. Gladys Berejiklian keeps reminding us that we are not out of the woods yet as far as COVID-19 is concerned and that disregarding public health orders over social distancing and hygiene regulations may ultimately put many of us at risk of contracting and spreading this disease.

It's interesting to note that there have been no significant changes in the COVID-19 case numbers attributed to those June long weekend mass rallies in the following months. If there was a substantial spike in COVID-19 infections attributed to the rallies only and not Australian citizens returning from overseas, then people may be extra concerned and take the contagiousness of this disease more seriously. As there were no new infections traced to the protest rallies, many people were left questioning the legitimacy of this pandemic and the mass chaos it has caused, both financially and socially.

Face masks

People refusing to wear masks is another form of social rebellion. There has been a lot of controversy around the wearing of masks and health agencies are not always in agreement with who needs to be wearing them and who doesn't.

In a scientific study, researchers set out to compare the efficacy of cloth masks with medical masks in hospital healthcare workers and concluded, 'This study is the first RCT [randomised controlled trial] of cloth masks, and the results caution against the use of cloth masks. This is an important finding to inform occupational health and safety. Moisture retention, reuse of cloth masks and poor filtration may result in increased risk of infection.'[65]

The authors of an editorial article in the *Journal of the American Medical Association* (JAMA) state, 'Cloth face coverings can substantially limit forward dispersion of exhaled respirations that contain potentially infectious respiratory particles in the 1 to 10 micrometre range that includes aerosol particles.'[66]

An issue with cloth masks is the minute size of the viral particles seeping through the weave of the cloth. The COVID-19 viral particles are very tiny at just 120 nanometres across.[67] This measurement converts to 0.12 of a micrometre and, to put this size in perspective, approximately 100 million viral particles would fit on the head of a pin.[68] As can be seen, COVID-19 virus particles at 0.12 micrometre in diameter are much smaller than the one to 10 micrometre viral particles referred to in the above *JAMA* article.

Dr Thomas Rainey, process engineer at the Queensland University of Technology, and his team have been working on developing a new highly breathable nanocellulose material that can remove particles smaller than 100 nanometres, a measurement in the range of viruses. The cellulose nanofiber material is made from waste plant material such as sugarcane bagasse and other agricultural waste products. It's biodegradable and can be easily manufactured for use as disposable filters in facemasks. 'This new material has excellent breathability,' said Dr Rainey, 'and greater ability to remove the smallest particles.'[69] Tests showed the new material had more breathability than commercial face masks, including surgical masks, and can be quickly made into large quantities using simple equipment. The material would be relatively inexpensive to produce and would therefore be suitable for single use. Dr Rainey and his team have established proof of concept as a nanoparticulate filtration material and are currently seeking industry partners.

Irrespective of the many different views on the efficacy of face masks, it's important to abide by local government mandates on this issue to avoid hefty fines, bearing in mind that medical masks are much more effective than cloth masks. The use of medical masks, however, depends on supply. When using any face covering, hygiene is very important. Medical masks should be replaced regularly and disposed of appropriately. If using cloth masks, they should be washed regularly and dried thoroughly before reuse.

International review

The Australian prime minister, Scott Morrison, has called for an independent global review into the cause of COVID-19, including China's handling of the initial outbreak in the city of Wuhan, in order to be better prepared for future pandemics. Our failure to carry out this investigation and proactively address this and other issues such as our relationship with China will almost certainly guarantee our failure to protect ourselves from similar or more deadly pathogenic outbreaks in the future. This inquiry, initiated by Australian Foreign Affairs Minister Marise Payne, was well-received by the international community.

At the 73rd World Health Assembly, the first-ever to be held virtually, delegates from more than 130 countries adopted a landmark resolution to unite and fight the COVID-19 pandemic. Specifically, WHO director-general, Dr Tedros Adhanom Ghebreyesus, called for 'an independent and comprehensive evaluation of the global response, including, but not limited to, WHO's performance.'[70]

Marise Payne has urged China to allow transparency in the process and added that she does not believe WHO should run the inquiry. This inquiry needs to be impartial, independent and comprehensive, she said. Jacinda Ardern, Prime Minister of New Zealand, is backing the inquiry, saying, 'We're not interested in blame; we're not interested in any kind of witch-hunt; we're just interested in learning.'[71] Local citizens are usually innocent victims; it's particular governments, regimes and institutions that need to be held accountable, especially where ethical issues and corruption are indicated.

The Chinese government has taken offence at the mere suggestion of this global inquiry and has retaliated by imposing an 80% tariff on Australian grown barley, suspending beef imports from four Australian abattoirs and suggesting that Chinese students would be reluctant to come to Australia for education because of concerns over racist incidents. The trade war between China and Australia has continued to escalate over time, with China stopping shipments of wine, copper, barley, coal, sugar, timber and live lobster.[72] Another retaliation has been a major cyberattack on the Australian Government and industry bodies seriously jeopardising our national security.

Scott Morrison said in a press conference at Parliament House, Canberra, on 19 June 2020, 'This activity is targeting Australian organisations across a range of sectors, including all levels of government, industry, political organisations, education, health, essential service providers and operators of other critical infrastructure.'[73] Experts have told the ABC that these cyber attacks are most likely being directed and initiated by China's premier intelligence agency, The Ministry of State Security (MSS), in retaliation for banning the Chinese telco Huawei from our 5G network, and have since been increasing in intensity.

It was announced on 10 July 2020 by WHO chief, Tedros Adhanom Ghebreyesus, that an independent committee, with former New Zealand prime minister, Helen Clark, serving as a co-chair, will be set up to launch an investigation into the handling of the coronavirus, including how the pandemic happened and the role WHO played in trying to prevent the spread of this disease. The WHO chief said in a briefing that the greatest threat was not the virus but, 'rather, it is the lack of leadership and solidarity at the global and national levels … it is time for a very honest reflection. All of us must look in the mirror—the World Health Organisation, every member state, all involved in the response. Everyone.'[74] While this is encouraging, it's hoped the panel members, to be chosen by the two co-chairs, Helen Clark and Liberian president, Ellen Johnson Sirleaf, both having served on the United Nations Development Program, will be impartial in their deliberations and that their findings will be trustworthy and credible. WHO is an agency of the United Nations and loyalties will have to be put aside for an honest appraisal of the situation.

An interim account of this investigation was due to be handed down in November 2020 with the final report to be presented in May 2021, but this has been delayed. The team was only allowed to commence their investigations in Wuhan China on 28 January 2021 due to Beijing's requirements to 'prepare' for their visit. One can only hope that when this report is finally handed down, it will be the truth. As will be seen in the next chapter, gain-of-function research poses considerable risk to humanity and it will be interesting to see if this is highlighted in the international review.

Australia's questioning of the official narrative offers us some hope in a world of fraudulent science, political manoeuvring and disinformation. Corruption will be brought to the fore if the evidence has not been destroyed, and this is good because then it can be addressed. We just have to be more alert to deception for political and financial gain and understand that things are not always what they seem. This can be achieved by becoming aware of hidden truths about the COVID-19 pandemic detailed in this book and similar volumes, such as the meticulously researched *Corona False Alarm? Facts and Figures*, by Dr Karina Reiss and Dr Sucharit Bhakdi.

Perspective can also be gained by choosing to listen to news programs and social media that offer more balanced content, rather than just a heavy focus on left-wing political propaganda promoting communist/fascist ideals and ideology. We can accept the popular narrative for what it is, but we don't have to blindly subscribe to it. Balance is key.

Key concepts
- COVID-19 was declared a pandemic by WHO on 11 March 2020
- Eighty-one percent of the population who develop this disease will have mild to moderate symptoms, 14% will have more severe symptoms and 5% will be critically ill, requiring hospital care
- Only 9% of hospitalised patients recorded no comorbidity—additional diseases such as heart disease, diabetes, obesity and hypertension
- The PCR test used to diagnose COVID-19 is not fit for purpose with up to 97% false positives
- An international review has been established to determine the cause of the COVID-19 pandemic

Pearl of wisdom

'You can fool all the people some of the time, and some of the people all the time, but you cannot fool all the people all the time.'

—Abraham Lincoln

CHAPTER 2

Caught Off-guard

It was the best of times, it was the worst of times

Home alone together

I arrived in Sydney from New Zealand on 22 March 2020 and, after stepping off the plane at the airport and proceeding through customs and immigration, I could tell that I was coming home to a different country. I made my way to the domestic departure terminal and, again, there wasn't the usual crowd rushing around looking for flight lounges or waiting patiently at luggage carousels. The shops were very quiet, even those selling coffee. How strange it all seemed. There was certainly a sense of tension in the air so thick you could almost cut it with a knife. I said goodbye to my travelling companions I'd met on the tour and we all went our separate ways to catch our various flights home and into compulsory self-isolation for two weeks.

There was panic everywhere and you could certainly feel the negative vibe. COVID-19 hit me with such dizzying force, metaphorically speaking, after my very pleasant holiday, that it seemed like I had to scurry for cover in the nearest hidey-hole I could find—the safety of my home.

What is this all about? I wondered when I'd regained some form of sensibility after my long flight home. It seemed like I'd been punched in the face as soon as I'd stepped off the plane. But was that punch designed to knock me out or wake me up?

Reflecting on this feeling, I concluded that, in reality, the 'punch-up' was a bit of both. I had been thinking quite a lot about the precarious state of our world affairs and how that had come to be. Why is there so much anger and division in the world, so much negativity, greed and control? It seems like everyone is out to grab whatever they can to benefit themselves, generally without any consideration for others. I was beginning to think that this 'disease' was the manifestation of our collective, less-than-desirable thought patterns.

I started thinking about the Taoist concepts of yin and yang and how everything is meant to be balanced in life to achieve harmony, and the world was not balanced. According to Chinese theory, yin and yang are two complementary energetic forces, active and passive, that exist in the universe. They are a balance of male and female energy in all things, both animate and inanimate. It's the concept of there being two sides to the same coin, opposites attract, night always turns into day, tides ebb and flow, the seasons follow each other and don't get stuck in the deep-freeze of winter. For every action, there is an equal and opposite reaction. It's the heartbeat of our Earth and it's what keeps our hearts beating. Without all these different aspects clinging together in unity, there wouldn't be a whole. All parts have their opposite counterparts that fit together in perfect harmony, except for when they get out of balance.

My friend Sharon asked me on the phone one day when I was in self-isolation if I really believed that thought creates reality.

'Yes,' I replied.

'Why?' she asked, 'I can't understand why you would think that. I can't just think about something, like a peanut butter sandwich, and have it instantly put in front of me.'

I tried to explain to my friend that everything in the universe is energy, beginning with thought, amplified by emotions and accelerated with action, and this includes fear.

After this conversation, I found myself thinking about fear and how it seemed to be surrounding us everywhere. I recalled being in fearful life-or-death situations before that had seemed all-consuming, and it was only when I'd educated myself about the process and attempted to understand the driving forces, that I'd been able to face them head-on and reduce a blazing fire of fear to a barely smouldering ember.

My fear-factor at the moment is low—enough that I am still on-guard, but I am certainly not running at a thousand miles an hour.

It's with this knowledge and understanding that I decided to educate myself as much as possible about the COVID-19 pandemic for the benefit of myself, my family and friends, and the wider community.

The political and medical landscape

We live in a rapidly changing and complex world and it seems that the democratic ways we once took for granted are being eroded by communist/fascist ideals and ideology and influenced by authoritarian governments. Our freedoms and liberties have been severely challenged, along with our privacy, as an ever-increasing number of measures are put in place to control us, dictating how we interact with others and live our lives.

Are we being primed for conquest and defeat by the dictates of authoritarian rule to force social change and mandate vaccines? Military personnel say that physical wars are no longer needed. Biological warfare with oppressive dictatorial measures seemingly works very well at controlling people in the world and invoking enough fear, at this point in time, to demand salvation in a syringe.

There is a lot we still don't know about this coronavirus and its origins. We do know that the SARS-CoV-2 outbreak started in China, as did the Avian Flu (H5N1) in 1997 and SARS in 2002, the Asian Flu in 1957 and despite its label, the Spanish Flu (H1N1) of 1918–1919 first appeared in China in 1917, according to some sources, exploding worldwide to kill between 20 and 50 million people. 'However, with no solid scientific evidence for the outbreak's cause, local Chinese health officials labelled it 'winter sickness' and chose not to quarantine citizens or enact travel restrictions.'[75]

The chair of the Australian Parliamentary Joint Committee on Intelligence and Security, Andrew Hastie said, 'The Chinese Communist Party must take responsibility for the virus that began inside their borders and work with the rest of the world to prevent it from happening again. We are simply asking for transparency and co-operation.'[76]

The Chinese government has repeatedly blocked efforts by world governments to investigate the viral outbreak, saying it's 'politically motivated'. They have also taken direct action to destroy evidence and arrest whistle-blowers such as the young Chinese ophthalmologist, Li Wenliang, who tried to warn the world of this dangerous viral outbreak and what was unfolding. Li Wenliang was summoned to the Public Security Bureau on 3 January 2020 and ordered to sign a letter claiming he had made false comments that had 'severely disturbed the social order'.[77] Li Wenliang subsequently died of COVID-19 on 7th February 2020, aged 34 years.

The Chinese regime delayed the mandatory reporting of this infectious outbreak to WHO and have been very adept at orchestrating misinformation and censorship campaigns to throw investigators and researchers off-target. 'We are fighting the virus at the moment, we are concentrating all our efforts in fighting against the virus,' said Chen Wen, a UK-based Chinese diplomat. 'Why talk about an investigation into this? This will divert not only attention; it will divert resources.'[78]

Can we trust politicians and health authorities?

The short answer is, apparently not. An editorial article was published in the *British Medical Journal* on 13 November 2020 with the headline, 'When good science is suppressed by the medical-political complex, people die'. In this explosive article, the author states, 'Science is being suppressed for political and financial gain. COVID-19 has unleashed state corruption on a grand scale, and it is harmful to public health. Politicians and industry are responsible for this opportunistic embezzlement. So too are scientists and health experts. The pandemic has revealed how the medical-political complex can be manipulated in an emergency—a time when it is even more important to safe-guard science.'[79]

The Great Reset versus the Great Awakening

There are two opposing battles currently underway in world politics—the Great Reset and the Great Awakening.

The Great Reset is a proposal by the World Economic Forum (WEF) to rebuild the economy sustainably following the COVID-19 pandemic focusing on climate change, sustainability, social justice and pandemic preparedness. It was unveiled in May 2020 by the United Kingdom's Prince Charles and WEF director Klaus Schwab.[80] Hailed as the 'Fourth Industrial Revolution', the Great Reset involves a transformation of society with permanent restrictions on fundamental liberties and mass surveillance by high-tech/big data giants, potentially using China's social credit system (discussed in chapter six), or something similar, to restrict democratic freedoms and temper 'wrongdoing'. Human beingness and enterprise will be changed forever with millions of people jobless. Goods and chattels will be sacrificed to the state in return for universal basic income. 'You'll own nothing and you'll be happy' is a frequently-cited phrase for a WEF 2030 prediction. If this prediction comes to fruition, AI will take over the world, mass vaccinations will control the population and basic necessities from online shopping will be delivered by drone.

The Great Reset has implications for food production where we will see 'farmerless farms being manned by driverless machines monitored by drones and doused with chemicals to produce commodity crops from patented GM seeds for industrial "biomatter" to be processed and constituted into something resembling food.'[81]

The reset has been referred to as a global plan to monitor

and control the world through digital surveillance.[82] It's 'a new "social contract" that ties every person to it through electronic ID linked to your bank account and health records, and a social credit ID that will end up dictating every facet of your life', according to the author of 'The Great Reset: What You Need to Know'.[83] It's described by some as an opportunity created by the chaos of COVID-19 and subsequent lockdowns to push through transformations that would not have been possible otherwise. It's an agenda to bring about global communism, or some might see it as communalism, and the complete enslavement of the human race all across the globe through the power of technology and the corrupt medical-political complex, as highlighted in the above articles. At a virtual meeting held in June 2020 hosted by the World Economic Forum, high-profile officials announced a proposal to reset the economy. 'Instead of traditional capitalism, the high-profile group said the world should adopt more socialistic policies, such as wealth taxes, additional regulations and massive Green New Deal-like government programs.'[84] Klaus Schwab said in 'What is the Great Reset?' referred to above, 'Every country, from the United States to China, must participate, and every industry, from oil and gas to tech, must be transformed.'

Many people are convinced that the Great Reset is a leftist movement designed to destroy free enterprise, free will, all private property rights such as home and farm ownership, as well as human rights such as freedom of speech, thought and beliefs and instead, we'll have tyrannical governments controlling all aspects of people's lives, land, labour, capital and resources. Rules, mandates and regulations will be enforced either by coercion or through the barrel of a gun, as intimated by Eric Worrall in his article 'What is the

Great Reset?' 'If the WEF Great Reset initiative succeeds, civilisation could end,' he said.

Alternatively, the Great Awakening and the end of an elitist era—people waking up to what is going on behind the scenes—is gaining momentum worldwide. This pro-liberty group rejects the media's deception and begins to see the world as it really is—good versus evil and the shades of grey in between.

People are beginning to understand that reality has been projected on them in a certain persuasive way by governments, institutions and the media to enforce a certain agenda, such as COVID-19 lockdowns and vaccinations, and this doesn't sit comfortably with their core beliefs or gut feelings. They are starting to believe that COVID-19 has been a smokescreen to usher in increased government and police powers to control people and strip them of their freedoms under the guise of draconian state of emergency laws. This smokescreen is becoming more transparent, and people are getting a glimpse of what a new dystopian future will look like—that persuasion is the first step towards tyranny, followed by coercion and then forced control.

The Great Awakening crusade is rising rapidly, countering the deep state socio-political corruption and the suppression of science to bring about a new beginning with a heightened awareness of the fragility of life in all its forms. This includes visionary measures to counter the human costs that have accompanied COVID-19—the economic collapse, social and physical losses and the dozens of new regulations that seem bent on keeping us apart. This cultural movement aims to build a new democratic society where social justice, human rights and ethical standards are respected, along with the intrinsic value of all human beings in an inclusive society.

As a society, we have come to a fork in the road and it's up to us as individuals to decide which path we wish to follow. What we have to decide, as a society, is if we want to embrace the dictatorship of communism or the liberty of democracy.

The World Health Organisation 'resets' its advice

Dr Maria Van Kerkhove, head of WHO's Emerging Diseases and Zoonoses Unit, said during a press briefing at the United Nations agency's Geneva headquarters on Monday 8 June 2020, 'From the data we have, it still seems to be rare that an asymptomatic person actually transmits onward to a secondary individual.'[85]

Dr Maria Van Kerkhove was forced to amend her comments the following day following criticism from epidemiologists across the world, saying 'asymptomatic spread is a "really complex question" and much is still unknown. "We don't actually have that answer yet".'[86] This is despite a scientific study published in the *Journal of Respiratory Medicine* clearly showing that when 455 people were exposed to an asymptomatic carrier of COVID-19, none of them contracted the disease.[87] It's no secret that highly-trained scientists are coerced to back-track or water down their scientific findings based on real data because their findings don't fit with a required political narrative, and if they don't, they suffer consequences.

The lack of asymptomatic spread has also been confirmed by a post-lockdown study of nearly 10 million residents in Wuhan, China, between 14 May 2020 and 1 June 2020.

The research paper, 'Post-lockdown SARS-CoV-2 nucleic acid screening in nearly ten million residents of Wuhan, China' was published in November 2020 in the scientific journal *Nature Communications*. The study was conducted by 19 scientists from China, Australia and the UK and it thoroughly debunked the concept of asymptomatic transmission.[88] Asymptomatic spread of SARS-CoV-2 has been the justification for worldwide lockdowns which have done nothing except hurt the most vulnerable in our community. The health and economic ravages of lockdowns have wrought unimaginable hardship, suffering and death on the masses while a few hundred billionaires have added to their massive fortunes in the greatest wealth transfer in history. The collective wealth of 651 billionaires in the US rose by $1.06 trillion (36%) in the nine months after the beginning of the pandemic,[89] while millions of working-class people have been forced to apply for unemployment benefits.

Medical experts worldwide have relied on WHO and other prominent health institutes to provide reliable medical facts and information to plan their responses to this pandemic which has resulted in lockdowns and isolating people in their homes, destroying economies, compromising lives and ruining livelihoods. This information has often been conflicting and misleading, which has added to the 'fear appeal' described in chapter three.

In a 2019 WHO report the authors indicate under the heading, 'Progress Indicator(s) by September 2020' page 10, 'The United Nations (including WHO) conducts at least two system-wide training and simulation exercises, including one for covering the deliberate release of a lethal respiratory pathogen.'[90] Bill Gates, co-chair of the Bill and Melinda Gates Foundation, and his friend and business associate, Dr Anthony Fauci, director of the American NIAID, both had an uncanny ability of being able to predict the Wuhan pandemic with 'astounding' accuracy. 'There is "no doubt" President Donald J Trump will be confronted with a surprise infectious disease outbreak during his term,'[91] said Dr Fauci.

Bill Gates also knew the pandemic was coming, even predicting it to start in a Chinese market in 2019, as disclosed in the Netflix documentary, *The Next Pandemic*.[92] Bill Gates has indicated that this is pandemic one and soon we will be experiencing pandemic two. 'Most of the work we are going to do is to be ready for pandemic two, I call this pandemic one,'[93] he said. Perhaps pandemic two will be the much-publicised second or subsequent wave which we are being cautioned about. Or perhaps pandemic two will be the highly infectious new mutated coronavirus strain now ravaging the United Kingdom and making its way around the world.[94] Perhaps this 'mutated coronavirus strain' is the result of the vaccine itself. Dr Fauci told a congressional committee on 12 May 2020, 'I must warn that there is a possibility of negative consequences where certain vaccines can actually enhance the negative effect of the infection'[95] through a phenomenon known as virus interference. 'In a viral video, virologist Dr Judy Mikovits says that a coronavirus vaccine could kill 50 million Americans in coming years, which will then be blamed on new strains of COVID, which will be used as a rationale for more, mandatory vaccines. The deaths will be due to viral interference which even Dr Anthony Fauci has warned of as problematic in vaccines.'[96]

Numerous scientists and doctors concede to threats, bribes and intimidation but some don't, such as Dr Judy

Mikovits, PhD, and others of similar integrity and moral courage who prioritise human life over business income. These are our heroes who have never wavered in their strong belief to uphold the truth, often at great personal and professional cost.

Many people believe that it is time for major reform—that WHO needs to stop acting as if it's a political organisation and start acting as a medical organisation. Medical facts should be promoted based on unadulterated science, not a political agenda to profit certain powerful individuals and institutions, such as patent owners and manufacturers of vaccines and ancillary supplies as well as big companies and businesses that have been allowed to trade normally at the expense of small to medium businesses, many of which were forced to close.

Foreign Affairs Minister and Senator, Marise Payne, is pushing for a reform of global bodies such as WHO and said, 'In the wake of this devastating health crisis, Australia wants to see a stronger WHO that is more independent and transparent.'[97]

Authoritarian Chinese Communist Party (CCP)

The CCP is hungry for power, emboldened by its vast economic and technological resources. Its authoritarian norms and tactics of intimidation and coercion have been exported on a massive scale worldwide resulting in an ideological struggle of 'cat and mouse' with the West. Every democracy is affected and their weaknesses are exploited for political gain.[98]

As more Western elites—governments, bureaucracies and business executives—become trapped in Beijing's economic stranglehold, the more they become afraid of Beijing's wrath if they don't tow the party line. One must not 'hurt the feelings of the people', with 'the people' meaning the party. Fear is being used as a weapon, and it's wielded mercilessly.

The extent of CCP influence, interference and subversion of Western democracies is beyond the scope of this manuscript, but an in-depth exploration of this subject can be found in the book *Hidden Hand: Exposing How the Chinese Communist Party is Reshaping the World*, by Clive Hamilton and Mareike Ohlberg. 'Democracies urgently need to become more resilient if they are able to survive,' say the authors of the abovementioned book. 'The CCP prefers to operate in the shadows [like white ants], and sunlight is often the best disinfectant ... Free speech and a free media are the enemies of the Chinese Communist Party and must be protected at all costs. Tantrum diplomacy and fear of economic retribution must not be allowed to prevent governments and others from calling out Beijing for its interference activities.'

China is developing its influence over the United Nations agencies and this is evident in the authoritarian style leadership we are currently experiencing. WHO is one of 15 agencies under the umbrella of the United Nations and four of these agencies are spearheaded by Chinese nationals. Foreign Minister Marise Payne said 'it was troubling that some countries were using the pandemic to undermine liberal democracy and promote their own, more authoritarian models'[99] and Russia and China have been instrumental in manipulating public debate.

WHO is coming under increasing scrutiny by truth seekers due to their inaction at the outset of this pandemic, promotion of disinformation and lack of transparency. The United States government was the largest sponsor of WHO but withdrew funding on 14 April 2020 and China stepped in to fill the void.[100] President Donald Trump has criticised WHO due to its close allegiance with China and its purported involvement in the 'escape' of COVID-19, unleashing havoc on the world.[101] Bill Gates, pro-vaccine advocate with personal pecuniary interests, is also a major sponsor of WHO and has had a lot to say about global health, unqualified as he is medically.

Gain-of-function research

Gain-of-function (GOF) research involves manipulating a pathogen in a laboratory, giving it extra properties or taking some away, that aims to increase its transmissibility and/or virulence. It can give a biological entity any new property and can speed up evolution.[102] 'Such research, when conducted by responsible scientists usually aims to improve understanding of disease-causing agents, their interaction with human hosts, and/or their potential to cause pandemics. The ultimate objective of such research is to better inform public health and preparedness efforts and/or development of medical countermeasures.'[103]

According to the US Department of Health and Human Services (HHS), GOF studies can not only improve the ability of a pathogen to cause disease but may entail biosafety and biosecurity risks. It's research that 'helps define the fundamental nature of human/pathogen interactions, thereby enabling assessment of the pandemic potential of emerging infectious agents.'[104]

Despite these potential benefits, GOF research can also pose substantial risks—it has dual-use potential, that of biodefense and biowarfare. It can be used for honourable purposes such as understanding viruses to prevent the next pandemic, or it can be used to 'generate biological agents with altered properties that enhance their weapon potential'.[101] High-security laboratory leaks are not uncommon and there have been a disturbing number of dual-use biodefense/biowarfare labs experiencing leaks, accidents and thefts over the past three decades.[105]

In 2014 the US Obama administration called for a pause in government funding for GOF experiments involving influenza, SARS and MERS viruses because of the high risk involved. Much of this research was carried out under the directorship of Dr Anthony Fauci at the NIAID and, when the US government paused funding, he moved his research to the Wuhan Institute of Virology and funded it through the EcoHealth Alliance by way of the National Institutes of Health in the US. Dr Shi Zhengli and other virologists in Wuhan studied bat coronaviruses extensively and used GOF research to alter their properties. In a 2008 article in the *Journal of Virology*, Dr Shi Zhengli and others report on how Chinese and US scientists have genetically engineered SARS-like viruses from horseshoe bats to enable the viruses to gain entry into human cells.[106]

On the 19 January 2018, United States Embassy scientists and diplomats met Dr Shi Zhengli, a virologist working at the Wuhan BSL4 laboratory, and sent warnings back to Washington about inadequate safety practices for research being conducted on bats and that the lab's work on bat coronaviruses and their potential human transmission represented a risk of a new SARS-like pandemic. 'During interactions with the scientists at the WIV [Wuhan Institute of Virology] laboratory, they [the scientists] noted the new lab has a serious shortage of appropriately trained technicians and investigators needed to safely operate this high-containment laboratory.'[107]

British ministers feared that a leak from a Chinese laboratory due to safety breaches may have caused the global pandemic. 'In 2018, the state-run *People's Daily* newspaper said the [Wuhan] laboratory is capable of conducting experiments with highly pathogenic microorganisms like the deadly Ebola virus. Experts from the institute were the first to suggest that the genome of the coronavirus was 96 percent similar to one commonly found in bats.'[108]

World politicians and intelligence agencies are now starting to believe that SARS-CoV-2 may have started as a benign bat coronavirus but was manipulated in a laboratory for GOF potential and escaped from the BSL4 lab in Wuhan. 'Right now, the ledger on the side of it leaking from the lab is packed with bullet points, and there's almost nothing on the other side.'[109]

The Chinese people were angry about what had happened. 'To make matters worse for leaders in Beijing, many Chinese [people] believe the virus either was deliberately released or accidentally escaped from the Wuhan Institute of Virology, a P4-level bio-safety facility,' said foreign affairs expert Gordon Chang in an opinion piece.[110] He went on further to say, 'China needs an enemy to blame because the Communist Party's inhumane and incompetent handling of the coronavirus outbreak has left many Chinese people white-hot angry.' The Chinese government might be blaming the US for this outbreak, but the Chinese people tell a different story.

Conspiracy theory or truth?

According to the *Encyclopedia Britannica*, a conspiracy theory is, 'An attempt to explain harmful or tragic events as the result of the actions of a small, powerful group. Such explanations reject the accepted narrative surrounding those events; indeed, the official version may be seen as further proof of the conspiracy.' It's often difficult to determine what is misinformation (conspiracy) versus legitimate information (truth), so how can you do it?

Critical thinking is a key skill in media and information literacy and people need to be able to question critically what they have read, heard and learnt. It's a matter of not simply accepting all arguments and conclusions you are exposed to but having an attitude involving questioning such arguments and conclusions. As mentioned previously, knowledge is important, but critical thinking is paramount when making the right decisions for ourselves and our wellbeing.

People are described as a conspiracy theorist when they reject the accepted narrative because it's not the truth as they have either experienced or seen with their critical thinking eyes. Many highly trained professionals have exposed their truth, but because it runs counter to the official narrative—what we are told to believe—these people have been slandered and all attempts have been made to destroy their credibility and evidence. Two such professionals are Dr Judy Mikovits, PhD, a highly trained virologist and author of the book, *Plague of Corruption: Restoring faith in the promise of science*, and retired US army sergeant and nurse, Erin Olszewski, who details her experiences as a frontline nurse working at Elmhurst, a COVID-19 public hospital in New York, treating mainly low socioeconomic patients. Erin's story can be viewed in her documentary film *Perspectives on the Pandemic*, episode nine, 'The (Undercover) Epicentre Nurse'.[111]

What is considered misinformation by some people at one point in time, may, in fact, become legitimate information sometime later. 'Coronavirus, which is killing and infecting people all over the world was created in a Lab in China's Wuhan, such an idea would have been labelled a conspiracy theory until a few weeks ago,' said Professor Giuseppe Tritto, an international expert in biotechnology and nanotechnology.[112] Professor Tritto, is also president of the World Academy of Biomedical Sciences and Technology, founded under UNESCO and has just released a book, *China COVID-19: The Chimera That Changed the World*, in which he insists the virus was genetically engineered and presents evidence to support that view.

According to Professor Tritto, the SARS-CoV-2 virus creation began after the 2003 SARS epidemic when Chinese researchers at the Wuhan Institute of Virology started working on a vaccine under the auspices of Shi Zhengli PhD, the scientist in charge of the program. 'Shi used reverse genetics to produce a SARS-like virus with increased pathogenicity with the help from the French Pasteur Institute, which showed her how to insert a segment from the HIV virus into a horseshoe bat coronavirus.' Tritto believes that although Shi Zhengli's research may have been initiated to develop a SARS vaccine, it progressed into a biological weapons effort using reverse genetics technology. Tritto also points out that as of September 2020, 11 different strains of SARS-COV-2 have been identified, making it extremely unlikely that a vaccine against this disease will be successful.[113]

Many other esteemed scientists and experts have also spoken out about the evidence for a laboratory origin of this disease. Andrew Kimbrell, executive director of the International Centre for Technology Assessment, states that SARS-CoV-2 is indisputably a chimeric (hybrid) virus because the bat coronaviruses that most closely resemble it do not have the same spike proteins and furin cleavage sites, allowing the virus access to human cells for reproduction and proliferation. Andrew Kimbrell notes, 'You have a basic bat coronavirus and you have two things that have been added to it. The spike protein is closest to an animal called the pangolin. We do know that somehow this bat virus was infected by at least two other animals and then went into a human host. And for that virus to be the way it is, it had to happen simultaneously ...'[114] He went on to say, 'Someone will have to come up with a scenario [for how that could happen]. It sounds almost like a joke. A horseshoe bat, a pangolin and some other creature met in a bar in Wuhan and somehow simultaneously infected them.'

Nikolai Petrovsky, professor of medicine and top vaccine researcher at Flinders University in Adelaide, Australia, said, 'The virus was not typical of a normal zoonotic infection since it appeared with the exceptional ability to enter human bodies from the beginning.'[115]

Whistle-blowers

Judy Mikovits, PhD

Dr Judy Mikovits PhD is a world-renowned immunologist and molecular biologist and has co-authored more than 50 peer-reviewed scientific papers. She was originally employed by Dr Fauci in 1980 as a postdoctoral scholar in molecular virology at the American National Cancer Institute and is a highly trained scientist. She also worked in top government laboratories on the Ebola disease, HIV and coronaviruses similar to SARS.

When she disclosed her research findings that conflicted with the agreed-upon narrative, she was ordered to cover up her data, but being a person of high moral principles, she refused to do so. She was threatened and sent to jail for five days with no charge other than an accusation of being 'a fugitive from justice'. Jail was a place where she was 'out of the way' so that her evidence could be located and destroyed, and this is all detailed in her book, *Plague of Corruption: Restoring faith in the promise of science.*

In the documentary video *Plandemic*, available at drjudymikovits.com, Dr Judy Mikovits is asked by the interviewer if she believed that this virus was created in a laboratory. She replied, 'I wouldn't use the word "created". But you can't say "naturally occurring" if it was by way of the laboratory. So, it's very clear this virus was manipulated. This family of viruses was manipulated and studied in a laboratory, where the animals were taken into the laboratory. And this is what was released, whether deliberate or not. That cannot be naturally occurring. Somebody didn't go to the market, get a bat. The virus didn't jump directly to humans. That's not how it works. That's accelerated viral evolution. If it was a natural occurrence, it would take up to 800 years to occur. This occurred from SARS1 within a decade. That's not naturally occurring.'

Dr Judy Mikovits' *Plandemic* video was banned on YouTube after receiving millions of views, but despite being banned, it has been launched on other platforms and has now hit one billion views worldwide, according to the *Australian National Review*, and has been described as 'the most viewed and banned documentary of all times.' A disclaimer for this controversial video at <u>drjudymikovits.com</u> says, 'This site exists to host *Plandemic*—a video that YouTube and other media giants have deemed inappropriate for you to view. We will not say whether or not we believe the video's allegations. We will say that there isn't a single corporation or government on this planet that has the right to decide what information we are allowed to receive.'

In another interview, Dr Mikovits said, 'There's a lot of data to support COVID-19 is not SARS-CoV-2 alone, and that it's SARS-CoV-2 and XMRVs, HGRVs and including human gammaretroviruses and HIVs.'[116]

Dr Mikovits is likely to be one of the most qualified scientists in the world to comment on this disease because of her ground-breaking research in molecular biology and virology, and yet we are being told what she is saying is 'nonsense' and that we should be listening to people like Bill Gates and his promise of vaccines, despite him having no medical training whatsoever! What he does have, however, is a conflict of interest—financial interests in vaccine production, giving billions of dollars in research funds in the name of philanthropy while at the same time expecting mega-profits in return.

Erin Olszewski

Erin is a retired army sergeant and nurse. *Undercover Epicentre Nurse: How fraud, negligence and greed led to unnecessary deaths at Elmhurst hospital* is the title of Erin Olszewski's new book released on 18 August 2020. Erin cared for COVID-19 patients in a private hospital in Florida and a public hospital in New York, and she witnessed a stark contrast in treatment protocols between the two facilities.

One of the treatment procedures for patients at the private hospital in Florida was hydroxychloroquine and zinc, and 'not one patient died' she said in her video.[117] This video was banned on YouTube after over one and a half million views but was made available at brighteon.com and other platforms. It is now available again on YouTube, at least for the time being. Dr Judy Mikovits' video was banned on YouTube too but is also available again now.

What Erin saw transpire at Elmhurst Hospital in Queens, a public hospital in New York catering for mainly low socio-economic patients, shocked her to the core. The management at Elmhurst purposely allowed COVID-19 transmission by placing COVID-19 positive patients alongside those testing negative. She observed how COVID-negative patients were listed as positive and placed on ventilation so the hospital could receive an extra $39,000 over and above other treatment expenses. Patients were denied CPR when circumstances were warranted and 'allowed' to die.

The CDC has identified that only six percent of coronavirus deaths are attributed to COVID-19 alone. Many patients with other diseases are being reclassified to bolster COVID-19 case numbers, for financial purposes in many instances. 'It has become policy in many hospitals to test for COVID-19 on admission. Patients coming in with severe chest pain are tested, even if they have no symptoms of the virus. Because of the CARES Act, there are plenty of financial incentives for them to list COVID-19 on the patient's chart—doing so results in higher levels of reimbursement at a time when hospitals are seeing less traffic due to fear of the virus. Early in the pandemic, some COVID-19 diagnoses were not even confirmed by tests. This led to a large-scale reclassification of deaths in places like New York.'[118]

Erin was not prepared to rest on her laurels about the human tragedy unfolding before her eyes at Elmhurst but chose to speak out about the injustices she observed by going undercover, recording conversations with other nurses and videoing instances of malpractice. Erin shared some of her observations in her video.

Appalled by how fraud, gross negligence, medical malpractice and greed led to unnecessary deaths at Elmhurst, Erin Olszewski has made it her mission to fight a new fight, not one of a physical, overt war with ballistics, as she'd been trained, but a more covert war in the medical field—one of a return to ethics, transparency and respect for the truth.

Human rights, social justice and ethics

Human rights are defined and protected by law and include basic rights and freedoms that belong to all people everywhere throughout their lifetime. These rights are based on shared values of dignity, fairness, equality, respect and independence, and include, but are not limited to, the right to equality, life, liberty and personal security, freedom from discrimination, torture and degrading treatment and the freedom of belief, opinion and information.

When a state of emergency is declared, such as with a pandemic, governments can restrict and suspend some rights temporarily to protect public health under human rights law. They also have the freedom to expand police powers, increase surveillance, close businesses and force people out of work. According to the United Nations High Commissioner for Human Rights, Michelle Bachelet, 'These restrictions need to be necessary, proportionate and non-discriminatory. They also need to be limited in duration and key safeguards against excesses must be put in place.'[119]

COVID-19 is not only a public health emergency but also an economic, social and emotional crisis that seems to be developing into a human rights crisis. Some governments and regimes have capitalised on the legality of 'exceptional measures', using them as a weapon to quash dissent, control the population and show themselves to the world as a powerful leader.

The city of Melbourne entered stage four lockdown on Sunday 2 August 2020 for six weeks due to an escalation in the number of COVID-19 cases. These restrictions included an overnight curfew where no one was allowed out of their homes between the hours of eight pm and five am unless they were leaving for medical care, caregiving or 'essential' work and were wearing a mask. No one was allowed to travel more than five kilometres from their home to exercise or shop. Exercise was limited to one hour per day either alone or in groups of no more than two. Only one family member was allowed to shop for groceries and food rationing for popular items was reinstated in some stores.

All non-essential shops, including most smaller retailers and sports complexes, were closed. Citizens who failed to abide by these rules faced a minimum fine of $1600.

It's all very well to have strong coronavirus measures to counter the spread of the disease, but there also needs to be strong oversight. Human rights advocates are urging federal and state governments to boost transparency and introduce safeguards to prevent the overreach of power. The coronavirus enforcement laws are a temporary measure during 'extraordinary circumstances' and need to be repealed when it's safe to do so. They are not to be used to 'play the people' and soften them up for a continuing political agenda, such as the enforcement of increased police powers, mandatory vaccinations and the introduction compulsory immunity passports to allow freedom of movement and participation in society.

The initial COVID-19 response in Australia was 14 days of self-isolation, which was expanded to four weeks in Melbourne and then six weeks. We were told it was necessary, just a little longer, just wear a mask, this might last for years, this is the new normal, all of which induce the three Ds: dependency, debility and dread—the pandemic creep! We don't want to find ourselves in a situation reminiscent of the boiling frog analogy, where we see our rights and liberties chipped away a little bit at a time until it's too late. The water in which we were comfortable becomes too hot and it's too late to jump out. We don't want to find ourselves relinquishing civil liberties and human rights for a false sense of security.

'Extraordinary times call for extraordinary measures,' said Australian Federal Treasurer Josh Frydenberg, but members of the Law Council of Australia started to question whether some of these 'extraordinary measures' became a little too extraordinary. Free speech, privacy, dignity and respect are human rights that have been sacrificed, in many cases, in the name of public health.

Antonio Guterres, Secretary-General of the United Nations, said, 'Human rights can and must guide COVID-19 response and recovery. The message is clear: People – and their rights – must be front and centre.'[120]

Professor Keith Scott-Mumby, who calls himself the official alternative doctor, has very strong views on this situation and said in his blog, 'This whole charade [about COVID-19] is a takeover of human rights that makes the Nazis and Khmer Rouge look like Red Cross volunteers.' He added, 'We are living in A WORLD GONE MAD. The whole health industry is on hold and dying as rapidly as patients. You can die of cancer, stroke, heart disease and diabetes. Nobody cares. But if you likely die of 'the virus', everyone flies into agonies of dread and threatens to return to lockdown, or even more wild measures for public safety.'[121]

In a United Nations publication, the authors state that given the exceptional situation and to preserve life, countries have had no choice but to adopt extraordinary measures to protect lives and livelihoods through extensive lockdowns, restricting freedom of movement and many other human rights. 'Such measures can inadvertently affect people's livelihoods and security, their access to health care (not only for COVID-19), to food, water and sanitation, work, education – as well as leisure.'[122]

Social justice is the notion that everyone deserves equal economic, political and social opportunities. If we are going to re-build a better society in the post-pandemic future based on shared values, rights and opportunities, we need to ask some serious questions about what kind of society we want that to be rather than leave it to the machinations of authoritarian power to decide for us. Public health and policy are based on value judgements and we see this being played out in our pandemic world now.

Healthcare professionals make life and death decisions in hospital settings over the allocation of resources, taking into consideration not only those who need those resources most but also who has the most likely chance of recovery. Women and children are forced to remain with their abusers due to social distancing and lockdown measures, our elderly people are locked away in nursing homes and, in many cases, dying alone because visitors are prohibited. People with disabilities are viewed as expendable when other health priorities take precedence. Suicides are skyrocketing.

This is the hidden cost of the pandemic, which is being largely ignored. For example, reports of domestic violence have spiked in many countries around the world with the onset of COVID-19. According to Harvard University epidemiological estimates, one in three women experienced intimate partner abuse before the pandemic.[123] In early April 2020, the United Nations secretary-general, Antonio Guterres advised of a horrifying surge in global domestic abuse linked to COVID-19 lockdowns with calls to helplines having doubled since the pandemic was declared the previous month.[124]

There is also 'The Lonely Crowd'. Prior to the pandemic in 2019, in a University of Michigan study on healthy aging, 34% of adults aged 50 to 80 years were identified as feeling lonely. Since the pandemic, 60% of older people reported a lack of companionship and 41% felt isolated.[125]

In a report compiled by a research team from the University of Sydney, the authors state, 'Under the optimistic 'best case' scenario, over the period 2020-2025 the model forecasts 19,878 suicide deaths [in Australia], an increase of at least 13.7%.'[126] These issues and others are discussed further under 'negative outcomes' in chapter five.

The ethics of ventilator use

Dr Agomoni Ganguli Mitra, Post-doctoral Research Fellow in Political Philosophy and Bioethics at the University of Muenster, Germany asks the question, 'Should ventilators be prioritised for those with no underlying health conditions to help ensure better survival rates? Or should people in greatest need take precedence?'[127] Or should ventilators even be used at all, as, from observations in Melbourne with the initial stage four lockdown and many people hospitalised, they appeared to be killing more people than they were saving? A study of New York's largest health system has found that a large percentage of patients placed on ventilators died. 'The study was based on Manhattan's Northwell Health network where the overall death rate from coronavirus is as high as 20%. When it came to patients who had to be placed on ventilators, the death rate rose to an alarming 88%.'[128] The rate was even worse for patients over 65 who were placed on ventilators, with only three percent of these patients surviving, according to this study. Men were particularly vulnerable.[129]

Aborted human foetal cells in vaccines

Ethical concerns should be front and centre in the race to develop a vaccine for COVID-19. Is it ethical to infect a volunteer patient with COVID-19 in the name of research to trial a vaccine? Should vaccination be made mandatory, forcing people to be vaccinated whether they object to it or not? How do you decide who should be vaccinated first when limited supplies are available? Should wealthier people and nations be allowed to monopolise supplies, creating a shortfall for underprivileged people?

A major ethical dilemma is should vaccines using human aborted foetal cells be used on the human population? This means injecting a patient with the DNA from another human being that can, apart from ethical issues, be potentially tumorigenic to the patient. One such example is the HEK-293 cell line–Human Embryonic Kidney cells from aborted babies. The number 293 is simply the number allocated to this cell line research by the scientist. A vaccine candidate against COVID-19, referred to as Ad5-nCoV, is currently in human clinical trials in Canada and contains the HEK293 cell line.[130] Another human cell line used in vaccine production is the PER.C6 cell line created from the retinal tissue of an 18-week gestation aborted foetus.

As of December 2020, more than 200 vaccine candidates against COVID-19 are either under development or in human trials around the world and two vaccines have received regulatory approval in the US and one in the UK. At least five COVID-19 vaccines or vaccine candidates are using human foetal cell lines, HEK-293 or PER.C6. 'Moderna, Oxford University / AstraZeneca, CanSino Biologics / Beijing Institute of Biotechnology, and

Inovio Pharmaceuticals, are using a human fetal kidney cell line called HEK-293 ... Additionally, Janssen, the pharmaceutical division of consumer product giant Johnson & Johnson, is using the human fetal cell line PER.C6 to develop its vaccine.'[131]

Vaccine ingredients

Before making an informed decision on vaccination, people may wish to check out the list of ingredients, otherwise known as excipients, in the vaccine solution. Excipients are the inactive substances that serve as the vehicle, or medium, for a drug or active substance. They are used to facilitate the manufacture and use of medicines and are necessary compounds in the formulation of some drugs.

It's useful to be aware of excipients in drugs and vaccines because some of them can cause harm. Some harmful excipients include formaldehyde, aluminium, polysorbate 80, natural rubber latex, MRC-5 human diploid cells (lung cells from an aborted baby) and monosodium glutamate.

The CDC Vaccine Excipient and Media Summary highlights the preservatives, adjuvants, stabilisers, cell culture materials, inactivating ingredients and antibiotics in different vaccines, including those containing human foetal cells.[132] The excipient toxicology can be viewed by going to a search engine and search ingredient + toxicity, or ingredient + MSDS (material safety data sheet).

Vaccine inserts are a good source for toxicology information, usually listed under item number 13, 'Nonclinical Toxicology'. For example, the Hepatitis A vaccine (Havrix) under item number 13.1 'Carcinogenesis, Mutagenesis, Impairment of Fertility', states, 'Havrix has

Jab No Pay"). In addition, it has raised the possibility of banning unvaccinated children from childcare centres ("No Jab No Play").'[135] The authors conclude, 'The evidence does not support a move to an increasingly mandatory approach that could only be delivered through paternalistic, coercive clinical practices.'

Lack of moral conscience and integrity

The debacle over the use of the inexpensive anti-malarial drug hydroxychloroquine is an example where good science has been corrupted to pave the way for new, more expensive, and therefore profitable, drugs such as remdesivir to treat COVID-19, and this is discussed in detail in chapter three. Hydroxychloroquine has been proven to be very effective in treating patients with COVID-19, especially when administered in the early stages of the disease and when combined with zinc and the antibiotic azithromycin.

Power, corruption and greed have become like a cancer on society throughout history where money has been worshipped like a god by some elitists, rather than being used as an honourable medium of exchange, as highlighted below.

Lao Tzu on lawlessness and disorder

Lao Tzu is credited with founding the philosophical system of Taoism. He was a record keeper in the court of the Chinese Zhou Dynasty of the sixth century BC where he was respected for his great wisdom. It's believed that he grew tired of life in the Zhou court because the warring states were constantly fighting each other for supremacy and nothing could be done to maintain law and order.

Lao Tzu was appalled by the power, greed and corruption he witnessed, so he decided to leave his kingdom on a water buffalo, dressed incognito as a farmer. He was recognised by the guard at the western border pass who beseeched him to write down his wisdom before he departed the kingdom. It is believed Lao Tzu wrote the *Tao Te Ching*, translated loosely as *The Way of Virtue*, in one night, after which he left his heritage behind and disappeared from history.

Jesus and the money changers

Jesus and his disciples travelled to Jerusalem to celebrate the feast of the Passover where thousands of pilgrims had gathered from all over the world. Money changers and merchants had set up shop in the temple, selling their wares, extracting a profit sometimes much greater than the law allowed, and this made Him angry. 'And they came to Jerusalem. And he entered the temple and began to drive out those who sold and those who bought in the temple, and he overturned the tables of the money-changers and the seats of those who sold pigeons. And he would not allow anyone to carry anything through the temple. And he was teaching them and saying to them, "Is it not written, 'My house shall be called a house of prayer for all the nations'? But you have made it a den of robbers.'" (Mark 11:15–17) English Standard Version.

Charles Dickens and the Reign of Terror

The setting for Charles Dickens' historic novel, *A Tale of Two Cities*, is the French Revolution during the Reign of Terror (1793–1794) when 17,000 people were officially executed and a further 10,000 died in prison or without a trial. In his opening paragraph of *A Tale of Two Cities*,

Charles Dickens said, 'It was the best of times, it was the worst of times, it was the age of wisdom, it was the age of foolishness, it was the epoch of belief, it was the epoch of incredulity, it was the season of light, it was the season of darkness, it was the spring of hope, it was the winter of despair, we had everything before us, we had nothing before us, we were all going direct to heaven, we were all going direct the other way—in short, the period was so far like the present period, that some of its nosiest authorities insisted on its being received, for good or for evil, in the superlative degree of comparison only.'

It is more about politics than health

The Washington Times reported, 'In fact, COVID-19 will go down as one of the political world's biggest, most shamefully overblown, overhyped, overly and irrationally inflated and outright deceptively flawed responses to a health matter in American history ... The facts are this: COVID-19 is a real disease that sickens some, proves fatal to others, mostly the elderly—and does nothing to the vast majority. That's it.'[136]

The lethality of COVID-19 was based on modelling that was, 'Catastrophically high in its estimations', according to Ivor Cummins in his YouTube video 'Viral Issue Crucial Update Sept 8th: The Science, Logic and Data Explained'. 'It was out by a factor of 15+ and that's what threw the world into turmoil,' he said, as discussed in the introduction.

Society has been utterly decimated as a result of this outrageously flawed modelling. Many people in nursing homes and some others with comorbidities have died, either with or from COVID-19, and that is tragic, but also tragic is the situation of vast numbers of people dying because of the unintended consequences of COVID-19—people not being diagnosed and treated for other fatal conditions such as cancer, heart disease, diabetes and mental health issues because they were either too scared to go to their regular medical practitioners, didn't want to 'catch COVID' in a hospital setting or services were simply not available because of the political hysteria created around this disease.

Ivor Cummins said in his abovementioned video, 'The epidemic in Europe largely ended around May, early June and now we are down to very low levels and this is entirely in line with the influenza epidemics in the past.' He also said in this video, what we are experiencing now is a 'casedemic', where we have hyper-testing with PCR and when you increase testing you find viral fragments from COVID-19 or other coronaviruses; dead virus from people who have recovered months ago and are asymptomatic. You will find some positive cases, but there will be very little impact. We have a 'casedemic' due to stringent, draconian measures based on PCR testing.

Ivor's words of warning, 'Get educated guys and gals—or keep your head in the sand while your errant leaders destroy society around you.'

The future is for us to decide

It appears the prestigious scientific journal *The Lancet* is conducting its own investigations into the origins of the SARS-CoV-2 outbreak with The Lancet COVID-19 Commission promising to 'leave no stone unturned'.[137] This investigation is being led by Dr Peter Daszak, who is a firm supporter of the natural evolution theory. But when we take a peek down the rabbit hole, we see conflicts of interests. Dr Daszak is president of the EcoHealth Alliance, which received funding from the NIH for GOF research to continue at the Wuhan Institute of Virology after the Obama administration paused funding for this research in 2014 when President Obama considered this research too risky.

If dangerous GOF research is to continue, it's imperative that the natural zoonotic origin of this coronavirus is preserved, otherwise 'it would shatter the scientific edifice top to bottom', as described by Antonio Regalado, biomedicine editor of *MIT Technology Review* in the abovementioned article.

If this research is allowed to continue, we will likely see and experience even more dangerous pathogenic pandemics in the future. As mentioned in the above article, 'Researchers at the University of Pittsburgh are looking to insert the SARS-CoV-2 spike protein, which is what allows the virus to gain entry into human cells, into Bacillus anthracis, the causative agent of anthrax, an already devastatingly dangerous pathogen.'

If the public remains uninformed, allowing the weaponisation of pathogens to continue unabated, it's possible that even more deadly consequences, medical and political, will be unleashed onto unsuspecting populations around the world. The public must become 'sufficiently aroused to demand real change', and that is part of the purpose of this book.

Key concepts
- Biological warfare replaces physical war
- CCP misinformation and censorship campaigns throw investigators off-target

- Viruses can be modified in a laboratory using GOF research. It speeds up evolution with potential to cause serious risk to biosecurity and biosafety and many laboratories have experienced leaks, accidents and thefts over the past three decades.
- The Obama administration paused GOF research funding in the US in 2014, but it was moved to the Wuhan Institute of Virology, where it continued
- US Embassy scientists met scientists at the Wuhan BSL4 laboratory and sent warnings back to Washington about inadequate safety practices

Pearl of wisdom

'The secret of freedom lies in educating people, whereas the secret of tyranny is in keeping them ignorant.'

—Maximilien Robespierre

PART 2

The Reaction: Treatments and Strategies

CHAPTER 3

Conventional Treatment

It was the season of light, it was the season of darkness

We can be like the sunflower

Before COVID-19 erupted onto the world stage, very few people were concerned about bioterrorism and its effect on national security, including health. A large portion of the general population hadn't even heard of coronavirus and most likely no one was harbouring any fears of a looming pandemic.

Global populations were going about their daily lives and things were predictable. We may have complained about unemployment, taxes, government action or inaction and climate change etc, but these contingencies were considered to be somewhat manageable, depending on who you spoke to.

Now our world has descended into chaos; things have changed, almost overnight. Some people are pinning their hopes on a vaccine to save the day, believing this is the only way we will be able to return to normal. Others are not confident that any vaccine produced will be safe and effective and are relying on measures such as optimising their vitamin D levels to manage this disease and learning to live with it if we have to.

When I asked one of my friends recently if she was going to have the vaccine, she said, 'Are you kidding? No, I am not going to allow anyone to inject me with a toxic cocktail of experimental poisons.'

Okay, I thought, *she has made her stance very clear*. When I asked another friend this same question, he said, 'Why would you *not* consider having it, it is the only way to protect ourselves and our future.'

There are also a lot of people who are undecided about this issue. They are 'sitting on the fence', waiting to see what happens to other people when vaccines are approved and administered to the general population.

What is important, I believe, is that we find the origins of this disease and deal with it to prevent similar or even more deadly pandemics in the future. If we don't, our coming years may be very bleak indeed and what we don't want is more of the same, or worse.

As citizens, we have a moral obligation to hand the baton, and the world, over to the next generation in better shape than what we experienced ourselves. World War I was supposed to be the war to end all wars but World War II followed 21 years later. After WWII, during the 1950s and '60s, industry and business boomed. We all had a bright future, at least in the Western world, if we were prepared to work hard for ourselves, our family and community.

When the post-war baby boomer generation came along, production and consumption increased, houses became bigger, people travelled more, disease was controlled, welfare and Medicare became available and most people lived fairly comfortable lifestyles. People had few genuine cares, other than those relating to their immediate needs and, generally speaking, life was quite good, at least on my home turf.

Migrants flocked to Australia in droves, loving our country down under. We had high employment, people worked hard and overseas students valued our education system. People enjoyed our laid-back lifestyle and leisure time in the sun, surf and sand, or around the barbeque. Our economy was strong and business was flourishing, but all that changed, seemingly overnight, and desperation set in.

The difference between hope and despair, I believe, is a person's attitude or outlook. I am reminded of Lao Tzu's quote from the second verse of the *Tao Te Ching*, 'So the sage lives openly with apparent duality and paradoxical unity' and we can be like 'the sage'.

Hope and despair may seem like opposites, but they are cut from the same cloth; without one we would not know the other. Despair colours the way we look at things in shades of grey. If we want to be happy, we have to accept life for what it is and let go of what we can't control. Hope springs eternal—it's human nature to keep on hoping against all odds like the sunflower plant does when engulfed in shadow—it turns its head relentlessly towards the sun. We can say to ourselves, 'I want to be like a sunflower so that even on the darkest days I will stand tall and find the light.'

Reflections

As we grapple with the fall-out of this pandemic, one thing is certain. This crisis has highlighted the weaknesses in our system. There needs to be a greater emphasis on health care and boosting our immune system, rather than focusing on sick care and treating symptoms. Prevention is better than cure; there is little to be gained from closing the stable door after the horse has bolted.

Our immune system is our bastion—our knight in shining armour—to defend us against sickness and disease, and it needs to be nurtured and protected at all costs. We need to promote agriculture and the purity of food; nutrition is key. We need to act quickly if and when we are caught in this situation again and, most importantly, we need to know the origins of this pandemic and how it started so we can prepare ourselves for the future.

We need to trust our gut feelings—think twice and act wisely. Will we be pandemic-wise in the future or politic-foolish? Will we learn from our mistakes, use our intuition and trust the process? Only time will tell.

Current treatment

Initially, there was no standard treatment for COVID-19 and symptoms were treated symptomatically. Many people who become ill are able to successfully recover at home with a treatment protocol similar to that of the flu, such as getting adequate rest, staying well-hydrated and taking over-the-counter medication to relieve fever, aches and pains. As time has progressed, other treatment protocols have become available for those more seriously affected such as monoclonal antibody therapy, convalescent plasma, the new antiviral drug remdesivir and the anti-inflammatory drug dexamethasone. Details of these treatments and procedures can be found at 'Treatments for COVID-19: What helps, what doesn't, and what's in the pipeline', authored by the Harvard Medical School, published March 2020 and updated November 2020. Other treatments discussed in this article include vitamin D, vitamin C, chloroquine, hydroxychloroquine and azithromycin. Intensive care is needed for complicated forms of the disease and non-invasive (NIV) and invasive mechanical ventilation (IMV) may be necessary in cases of respiratory failure refractory to oxygen therapy.

The race for a vaccine

There are two mantras that we commonly hear, 'We are all in this together,' and 'the race for a vaccine.' As of 22 December 2020, more than 200 coronavirus vaccines are being developed across the world, according to WHO.[138] The US government's Operation Warp Speed initiative has pledged $10 billion to develop and deliver 300 million doses by January 2021 and WHO is aiming to deliver two billion doses by the end of 2021.[139] As stated in this article, it normally takes 10–15 years to bring an effective vaccine safely to market, but clinical processes are being compressed in the name of urgency.

And the winner is Pfizer/BioNTech

The Pfizer/BioNTech mRNA vaccine candidate is the first to be authorised in the Western world for emergency use with the United Kingdom paving the way. The UK health regulator announced on 2 December that this vaccine had passed the necessary regulatory approval for emergency use and a 91-year-old grandmother, Margaret Keenan, was the first to receive a jab on 8 December 2020 as an early birthday present. An additional 800,000 doses will be dispensed in the coming weeks with up to another four million by the end of December 2020.[140] Operation Warp Speed—in less than a month after receiving regulatory approval, Pfizer/ BioNTech will have been able to manufacture almost five million doses of their vaccine and have it available to the public!

On 9 December 2020, *The New Daily* reported that the US FDA revealed six people died in Pfizer's late-stage trial just after Britain rolled out the vaccine, 'but the deaths are said to raise no new safety issues or questions about the vaccine's effectiveness.'[141] On 10 December 2020, the UK's medicine regulator issued a warning for anyone with a history of anaphylaxis to a medicine or food not to get this vaccine.[142]

Two mRNA vaccines receive FDA approval

Two vaccine treatments have recently been approved by the FDA for use in the US with those being the Pfizer/ BioNTech candidate approved on 11 December 2020 and the Moderna/NIH vaccine receiving the tick of approval on 18 December 2020. Both of these authorisations are initially for emergency use only with front-line health workers and vulnerable people receiving priority. These two vaccines contain messenger RNA (mRNA) which is genetic material that instructs cells in the human body to make the SARS-CoV-2 spike protein normally found on the surface of coronavirus cells.

It's anticipated that the non-infectious COVID-19 spike

proteins produced by the body after vaccination in the form of protruding spikes and protein fragments, will encourage the immune system to produce antibodies, lock onto an invader virus, mark it for destruction and thus prevent the virus from entering human cells via the ACE2 receptors.[143] The ACE2 receptors have other important functions such as offering protection against cardiovascular, lung and kidney diseases.[144] 'Women have two copies of the ACE2 gene and men only have one copy,' Professor Gavin Oudit said in this article. 'This does not seem to make women more susceptible to COVID-19 infection, but it does protect them from the complications associated with the virus.'

Robin Shattock, Professor of Mucosal Infection and Immunity at the Faculty of Medicine, Imperial College London, and his team 'are convinced that the presence of viral spikes alone will be enough to wake up the immune system and produce an antibody response. Once your body has "learnt" to recognise that these viral spikes are foreign and need to be swamped by neutralising antibodies, it will be in a better position to rapidly respond when it encounters a real virus covered in the same spikes.'[145]

Pfizer and Moderna mRNA vaccines reported to be 95% effective

These two pharmaceutical companies are reporting very impressive results with their mRNA vaccines in the vicinity of being 95% effective. This is a massive feat considering no previous vaccine in history has ever come close to this level of effectiveness despite huge budgets and many years of research. And no successful coronavirus vaccine has ever been produced before! Ross Walter, Nutritionist and Naturopath, explained how they arrived at their effectiveness percentage. 'Allegedly, Pfizer is testing their mRNA vaccine on 44,000 volunteers. They reported 170 COVID-19 cases in the volunteers, with 162 in the placebo group and 8 in the vaccine group. They get their 95% effectiveness by comparing the COVID cases between the placebo group against the vaccine group, as (8/162) * 100% = 4.9% or rounded up to 5% COVID cases in the vaccinated group compared to 95% in the non-vaccinated group. Therefore, they say their vaccine is 95% effective!'[146]

Dr Niran Al-Agba, a paediatrician in Silverdale, Washington, has a similar explanation for how the numbers are derived. Pfizer recruited 43,661 healthy volunteers for their trial with half of them to receive the 'experimental' vaccine and the other half the 'placebo', which is normal protocol. 'Researchers waited until 170 people going about their normal activities, tested positive for COVID-19. Out of those who contracted COVID-19, 162 received the placebo shot, while 8 received the experimental vaccine, yet still became infected. If a vaccine had 100% efficacy, no volunteers given experimental vaccine would get COVID-19. Since 8 did, efficacy is reported at 95%.'[147]

Moderna has used the same testing criteria as Pfizer with approximately equal effectiveness. However, there's a huge difference between relative risk reduction and absolute risk reduction. In the article 'Side Effects and Data Gaps Raise Questions on COVID Vaccine', Dr Mercola comments, 'While Pfizer claims its vaccine is 95% effective, this is the relative risk reduction. The absolute risk reduction is actually less than 1%. This is the typical Big Pharma trick: confusing absolute and relative risks ... Analysis of recently released data suggests the relative risk reduction for Pfizer's vaccine may actually be between 19% and 29% – far lower than the licensing threshold of 50%.'[148] Peter Doshi, Associate Editor of the *British Medical Journal* said, 'There may be much more complexity to the "95% effective" announcement than meets the eye—or perhaps not. Only full transparency and rigorous scrutiny of the data will allow for informed decision making. The data must be made public.'[149]

Australia won't automatically follow the UK and US, with Prime Minister Scott Morrison saying on 11 December 2020 at a National Cabinet Meeting, 'On the issue of accreditation approval of vaccines in Australia, we will do that on Australian rules with Australian officials and on the Australian timetable.'[150]

Further details in relation to vaccines are discussed later in this chapter.

Remdesivir

Remdesivir, sold under the brand name Veklury by Gilead Biosciences, was originally a drug developed to treat Ebola. It has received provisional approval in Australia as a treatment option for patients hospitalised with severe COVID-19 infections. It's not available for people in the general community because it can cause severe side effects which need to be monitored closely. In a study conducted in France on five hospitalised COVID-19 patients treated with remdesivir on compassionate grounds, researchers reported, 'The cases of the five patients presented herein highlight some difficulties with remdesivir infusion when administered in most patients with advanced disease. Particular attention should be paid to hepatic and kidney function when administering this treatment.'[151]

Deputy Chief Health Officer, Nick Coatsworth, said in a *Sydney Morning Herald* article, that remdesivir is not a 'silver bullet' but may have effects that 'include a reduction in the length of hospital stay, and a potential reduction in the serious adverse events that coronavirus sufferers can get during their episode of coronavirus disease'.[152] He also said, 'What we don't know yet is whether it has a conclusive effect on mortality.' In a study published by *The Lancet*, the authors conclude, 'In this study of adult patients admitted to hospital for severe COVID-19, remdesivir was not associated with statistically significant clinical benefits.'[153]

Dr Hugh Cassiere is the director of critical care services for the Sandra Atlas Bass Heart Hospital in Manhasset, Long Island, and he commented in a video that remdesivir is 'not the blockbuster that we thought it was going to be … I would recommend remdesivir early, early on in the disease.' When reflecting on what he learnt treating patients with COVID-19 over the last few months, he said, 'If I can go into a time machine and go back to March 14, 2020, I would tell myself the day before start using steroids freely, dexamethasone, on all your critically unstable COVID-19 patients.' Dexamethasone is a steroid medication that reduces inflammation. Dr Cassiere also said, 'It's the only therapy that's been shown to save lives … everything else is more supportive therapy.'[154] He went on further to say, 'According to a University of Oxford study, dexamethasone reduced the mortality rate of patients on ventilators by one-third. The mortality rate for patients requiring only oxygen was cut by one-fifth.'

A representative from the Australian Therapeutic Goods Association (TGA) said in an *ABC News* report, 'While this is a major milestone in Australia's struggle against the pandemic, it is important to emphasise that the product has not been shown to prevent coronavirus infection or relieve milder cases of infection.'[155] Remdesivir is expensive and, 'it is the only drug to have been licensed by the US and the European Union as a treatment for severely ill coronavirus patients', according to this news report. It will be subsidised for use in Australia by the government when donated supplies from the manufacturer are extinguished. Victoria's Chief Health Officer, Brett Sutton said, 'While the Australian government would try to secure its own supply, stocks were affected because the "US really went very hard in gobbling up the entire global supply".'[156]

There are obviously conflicting statements on the use and efficacy of remdesivir and the target group it is recommended for. Caution is warranted.

Dexamethasone

The anti-inflammatory drug dexamethasone, a steroid, has also been approved for use in Australia. It's a cheap drug that has been around since the 1950s and has been used to treat a range of conditions related to inflammation such as severe allergies, arthritis and asthma. It's recommended for hospitalised patients with severe COVID-19 infections in both Australia and the United Kingdom.

WHO has welcomed positive preliminary results with Dr Tedros Adhanom Ghebreyesus, WHO Director-General, stating in a news release, 'This is the first treatment to be shown to reduce mortality in patients with COVID-19 requiring oxygen or ventilator support. ... This is great news and I congratulate the Government of the UK, the

University of Oxford, and the many hospitals and patients in the UK who have contributed to this lifesaving scientific breakthrough.'[157] WHO further commented in this news release, 'Dexamethasone, a corticosteroid, can be lifesaving for patients who are critically ill with COVID-19. For patients on ventilators, the treatment was shown to reduce mortality by about one third, and for patients requiring only oxygen, mortality was cut by about one fifth, according to preliminary findings.'

Hydroxychloroquine and chloroquine

There has been a lot of controversy over the use of hydroxychloroquine and chloroquine in the treatment of COVID-19 which, unfortunately, has become a political football. Both chloroquine, and its milder derivative, hydroxychloroquine, are inexpensive anti-malarial drugs with the former developed in 1934 to treat malaria and the latter, an analogue of chloroquine, was developed in 1946 to treat autoimmune diseases such as systemic lupus erythematosus (SLE) and rheumatoid arthritis.[158] As stated in this article, 'In general, hydroxychloroquine has fewer and less severe toxicities ... and fewer drug interactions than chloroquine,' in relation to treating malaria and autoimmune diseases.

In a news release issued by the US National Institutes of Health, the official narrative for the discontinuation of the use of hydroxychloroquine is, 'A clinical trial to evaluate the safety and effectiveness of hydroxychloroquine for the treatment of adults hospitalised with coronavirus disease 2019 (COVID-19) has been stopped by the National Institutes of Health. A data and safety monitoring board (DSMB) met late Friday and determined that while there was no harm, the study drug was very unlikely to be beneficial to hospitalised patients with COVID-19.'[159]

Dr Anthony Fauci joined the US NIH in 1968 as a clinical associate in the Laboratory of Clinical Investigation (LCI) at NIAID. In 1984 he became director of the NIAID and was appointed one of the lead members of the Trump administration's White House Coronavirus Task Force. The NIH recommended against the use of chloroquine or hydroxychloroquine with or without azithromycin for the treatment of COVID-19, except in a clinical trial.[160] This stance has been adopted by WHO, a specialised agency of the United Nations responsible for international public health and from which world health authorities in various countries seek advice.

Chloroquine is a potent inhibitor of SARS coronavirus infection and spread

The NIH comprises 27 separate institutes and centres and the NIAID comes under this umbrella. The *Virology Journal* is an official publication of the NIH. A research article, 'Chloroquine is a potent inhibitor of SARS coronavirus infection and spread', dated 22 August 2005, was published in the *Virology Journal* when Dr Fauci was the director of the NIAID. The results of this study clearly state:

> 'We report, however, that chloroquine has strong antiviral effects on SARS-CoV infection of primate cells. These inhibitory effects are observed when the cells are treated with the drug either before or after exposure to the virus, suggesting both prophylactic [prevention] and therapeutic [treatment] advantage.'[161]

Dr Fauci would have known of the effectiveness of chloroquine in treating SARS-CoV-1 and the potential for hydroxychloroquine as an effective treatment for SARS-CoV-2 given that these diseases are genetically related. SARS-CoV-2 shares 79% of the genome of SARS-CoV-1.[162]

The NIH and WHO recommend the use of the expensive remdesivir drug for COVID-19 patients with severe infections being treated in hospital, prioritising the patients who receive it due to limited supplies.

As of 11 August 2020, Dr Fauci is no longer President Donald Trump's key advisor on the White House Coronavirus Task Force, having been sidelined by the hiring of Dr Scott Atlas, a former Stanford University Medical Centre chief of neuroradiology. As head of the NIAID, Dr Fauci still has a central role in the management of the pandemic, together with Dr Robert Redfield, head of the CDC. 'Both the NIAID and the CDC are corrupt entities. A relentless fear campaign is ongoing sustained by fake data and manipulated death certificates.'[163]

Dr Atlas had a more conservative view and 'warns against coronavirus overreaction and hysteria'. He went on to say, 'The fear campaign must be ended. It is based on lies and fabrications. Censorship of medical doctors should also be addressed.'

Jeff Zients has been appointed coordinator of President Biden's COVID-19 task force, despite him having no scientific or medical background, but this former consultant and entrepreneur has the confidence of his contemporaries to 'fix the mess left behind by the Trump administration'.[164]

Using hydroxychloroquine with zinc will end the COVID-19 plague

It was discovered that hydroxychloroquine is an effective antidote for COVID-19, especially when combined with zinc and the antibiotic azithromycin. Dr Vladimir Zelenko had treated over 900 COVID-19 patients up to 7 April 2020 with hydroxychloroquine sulphate, zinc and azithromycin with a very high success rate. His approach is to treat patients early so they don't have to be put on ventilators. 'My data will show that if you initiate treatment within the first five days, you have an 85% reduction in death and hospitalisation. What that means is that this infection becomes no different than any other infection' and that 'this medication, when scaled globally, will end this plague.'[165]

Hydroxychloroquine and zinc protocol

Dr Zelenko's successful treatment protocol is outlined in the abovementioned article. He was censored by the medical mafia, ridiculed and shamed. When asked in the video of the article referred to above why there is such resistance to the use of hydroxychloroquine, he commented, 'I can give you reasons why there's resistance. It's very simple, it's called politics, profit, arrogance and fear.'

Dr Zelenko now feels somewhat vindicated by a new study conducted by a team at the Henry Ford Health System in southeast Michigan and published in the *International Journal of Infectious Diseases*. This research was conducted on 2,541 hospitalised patients and it was found those given hydroxychloroquine were less likely to die. The conclusion of this study states, 'In this multi-hospital assessment, when controlling for COVID-19 risk factors, treatment with hydroxychloroquine alone and in combination with azithromycin was associated with reduction in COVID-19 associated mortality.'[166] 'Twenty-six percent of those not given hydroxychloroquine died, compared to 13% of those who got the drug.'[167]

It has been claimed many times that it's important to treat people with hydroxychloroquine in the early stages of the disease for maximum effectiveness, ideally before they become so ill that they need to be hospitalised. It's interesting, but not surprising, that zinc was not included in this clinical research. One day the conventional and natural therapies may rise above the tug-of-war duality of right and wrong and embrace more holistic and effective remedies for the health of people of all nations.

Despite this and other reported successes using the hydroxychloroquine protocol, this treatment has been discredited by the mainstream medical fraternity. When the question of hydroxychloroquine efficacy was discussed at a press conference, Dr Fauci said in a video it is purely anecdotal, and doctors and hospitals were forbidden to use it.[168] This is despite chloroquine, closely related to hydroxychloroquine, being scientifically proven to provide both prophylactic and therapeutic advantage in research published in the *Virology Journal*, 22 August 2005, as previously mentioned.

A study of the use of hydroxychloroquine or chloroquine for the treatment of COVID-19 appeared in *The Lancet* on 22 May 2020 and the *New England Journal of Medicine*, a short time later concluding, 'Each of these drug regimens was associated with decreased in-hospital survival and an increased frequency of ventricular arrhythmias when used for treatment of COVID-19.'[169] As a result of this multinational study, governments around the world have warned against using hydroxychloroquine for treating or preventing COVID-19, highlighting the drug's potential toxic side effects. This study was subsequently retracted because the science was corrupt. In an open letter to *The Lancet* written on 29 May 2020 and signed by 120 researchers and medical professionals from around the world, including Australia, serious concerns were raised about the statistical analysis and data integrity of the study. The data collected from Australia was not compatible with government reports, there was no ethics review and the statistical modelling was highly questionable.

It appears that Big Pharma and its medical minions organised a team of doctors to write this journal article to discredit hydroxychloroquine—an inexpensive, off-patent drug that has been available for 65 years to treat illnesses such as lupus, malaria and rheumatoid arthritis and officially labelled as safe, to pave the way for much more lucrative drugs such as remdesivir, from which fortunes will be made if approved for general treatment. Government lackeys are desperately trying to suppress information about natural and available cures, and integrative treatments that may eliminate COVID-19 before profitable vaccines and other pharmaceuticals can be made available to the general public.

One of the medical authors of 'Hydroxychloroquine or chloroquine with or without a macrolide for treatment of COVID-19: a multinational registry analysis' mentioned above, was supposedly the science editor of a bogus company called Surgisphere that purportedly had access to large amounts of de-identified data from a massive health care data analytics platform, including that of 96,000 patients in 1200 hospitals around the world, for the purpose of research. The actual cooperation of hospitals in Melbourne and Sydney was essential for the Australian patient numbers in the study.

When contacted by *The Guardian* Australia, all hospitals denied any knowledge of Surgisphere and disavowed any role in a database. It turns out that the 'science editor' of this fantasy research company is a part-time science-fiction author and an adult content model! Surgisphere is nothing more than a bogus front that invents data to be used by Big Pharma to discredit inexpensive off-patent drugs in order to put the media spotlight on high-profit pharmaceutical drugs and vaccines.

While many doctors have had success using hydroxychloroquine on its own to treat COVID-19, it works much better when combined with zinc and the antibiotic azithromycin. One of the primary effects of hydroxychloroquine is to increase the pH in the cell, making it more alkaline, at a specific point where coronaviruses replicate. Another effect is that it acts as an ionophore for zinc, meaning that it helps to transport zinc across the fatty cell membranes allowing access for zinc to do its magic as an anti-viral mineral. To a large extent, in this process, it's zinc that facilitates treatment. Other ionophores that carry out the same function as hydroxychloroquine, but at a reduced capacity, are the natural substances quercetin, a readily available nutritional supplement, and EGCG, an extract found in green tea.

This study of hydroxychloroquine is just one example of how populations and governments around the world have been duped. The definition of democracy, government of the people, by the people, for the people; the words of former US President, Abraham Lincoln, seems to have vaporised into thin air as corporate governments work with policies, not laws, that apply only to members of political parties and the public service to achieve a prescribed agenda.

Ivermectin

Ivermectin is an antiparasitic drug with an excellent safety profile that has been used to treat several tropical diseases. It is also very effective in providing prophylaxis (prevention) and treatment for COVID-19, according to Pierre Kory, M.D., Associate Professor of Medicine at St Luke's Medical Centre, a private hospital in Milwaukee, Wisconsin. In a YouTube video, this highly trained medical professional said, 'We have a solution to this crisis. There is a drug that is proving to be of miraculous impact … a scientific recommendation based on mountains of data that has emerged in the last three months showing the miraculous effectiveness of Ivermectin. It basically obliterates transmission of this virus. If you take it you will not get sick.'[170] This was part of Dr Kory's passionate testimony during the Senate Homeland Security and Governmental Affairs Committee hearing on 'Early Outpatient Treatment: An Essential Part of a COVID-19 Solution, Part II'.[171]

Several studies have been undertaken on the efficacy of ivermectin in preventing and treating COVID-19. This anti-parasitic drug has been shown to, '… inhibit the replication of many viruses … has potent anti-inflammatory properties … diminishes viral load … prevents transmission … hastens recovery … [and] leads to far lower case fatality rates in regions with widespread use.'[172]

Type I Interferons

Type I interferons, interferons alpha and beta, are signalling proteins and part of the innate immune response to viral infections. Different mucosal surfaces in the human body make type I interferons (IFN-I) and their role is to shut down the replication of RNA viruses such as coronaviruses and retroviruses early in the disease process. The natural production of interferons in the human body diminishes with age and a depletion in nutrient status.

Interferons can be manufactured by pharmaceutical companies and made available for the treatment of disease and researchers have concluded that type I interferon beta may account for a safe and easy-to-upscale treatment against COVID-19 in the early stages of infection. In vitro studies suggest that SARS-CoV-2 could be substantially more sensitive to IFN-I than other coronaviruses, such as MERS-CoV and SARS-CoV.[173]

The researchers of this study also said, 'The current lack of animal model for COVID-19 should not prevent the clinical evaluation of IFN-I treatment, since its safety has already been assessed in numerous independent clinical trials.' Scientists in China performed clinical trials of type I interferon treatment in early 2020 for COVID-19 and publication of that data should give more accurate information as to the relevance of this treatment.

Dr Judy Mikovits said that immune disruption with COVID-19 would be stopped with type I interferon alpha at a very low dose. She commented that it's possible to make a safe vaccine by putting a type I interferon at a very low dose, 50–200 units, in a capsule. When Merck made interferon, it was produced in a 50-million-unit vial costing approximately $600. 'That would provide 1000 people with two doses a day at 50–200 units, costing 50 cents a dose for a week.'[174]

Vitamin C is an essential antioxidant and enzymatic co-factor for many physiological reactions and will increase the production of interferons in the body to fight viral infections in the early stages of disease. 'Vitamin C exerts its antiviral properties by supporting lymphocyte activity, increasing interferon-α production, modulating cytokines, reducing inflammation, improving endothelial dysfunction, and restoring mitochondrial function.'[175] The benefits of quercetin and vitamin C will be discussed further in the following chapter.

More on vaccines—Oxford University/AstraZeneca

The Oxford University vaccine candidate AZD1222, made from a virus ChAdOx1 in partnership with the global pharmaceutical firm AstraZeneca, began phase III clinical trials in Brazil on 28 June 2020 with 5000 volunteers and aiming to recruit up to 50,000 volunteers in the United Kingdom, the United States and South Africa.[176] The aim of this study is '… [to] assess how well the vaccine works to prevent people from becoming infected and unwell with COVID-19.'[177]

The Oxford/AstraZeneca coronavirus phase III vaccine trials were paused in early September 2020 after a study participant suffered a serious adverse reaction[178] but resumed a few days later in the United Kingdom after the Medicines Health Regulatory Authority (MHRA) confirmed that the trials were safe to proceed. A press release from AstraZeneca stated that AstraZeneca and the University of Oxford 'cannot disclose further medical information' regarding the adverse event.[179]

Unlike the mRNA vaccines, designed to produce neutralising antibodies directed at a portion of the coronavirus 'spike' protein, the Oxford University candidate vaccine is made from a chimpanzee adenovirus called ChAdOx1 that has been genetically modified, making it impossible to grow in humans. It does, however, contain the active genetic material of the SARS-CoV-2 virus spike protein. 'After vaccination, the surface spike protein is produced, priming the immune system to attack the SARS-CoV-2 virus if it later infects the body', as reported in the abovementioned press release.

In the article 'AZD1222 SARS-CoV-2 Vaccine', the author describes how the SARS-CoV-2 coronavirus uses its spike protein to bind to enzymes called ACE2 receptors on human cells to gain entry to the cells and cause infection. 'By vaccinating with AZD1222 (ChAdOx1 nCoV-19), these researchers are hoping to make the body recognise and develop an immune response to the spike protein that will help stop the SARS-CoV-2 virus from entering human cells and therefore prevent infection.'[180]

Australian Federal Health Minister, Greg Hunt, said that the pause of the Oxford University vaccine trials will not prevent Australia from accessing the jab early in 2021.[181]

Risk versus benefit

For further clarification on the different types of vaccines, whether inactivated or attenuated whole virus vaccines, protein vaccines, viral vectors as gene-based vaccines and gene-based vaccines, please refer to chapter seven, 'Is vaccination the universal remedy?' in the book *Corona False*

Alarm? Facts and Figures by Dr Karina Reiss and Dr Sucharit Bhakdi, published by Chelsea Green Publishing, London, UK (2020). In this chapter under the heading 'To vaccinate or not to vaccinate, that is the question', the authors state in relation to gene-based vaccines, 'A great potential danger of DNA-based vaccines is the integration of plasmid DNA into the cell genome. Insertional mutagenesis occurs rarely but can become a realistic danger when the number of events is very large, i.e., as in mass vaccination of a population. **If insertion occurs in cells of the reproductive system, the altered genetic information will be transmitted from mother to child**' [emphasis added].

If individuals are vaccinated with the mRNA vaccines, such as the Pfizer and Moderna candidates, and their immune systems are unable to process the waste products naturally produced, they can potentially experience autoimmune attacks that are 'simply terrifying', according to the authors of the abovementioned book.

"Vaccine will only sterilize 70 per cent of the population"

The above statement was made by Sir John Bell, regius professor of medicine at Oxford University. He commented in a video on YouTube and elsewhere, 'These [COVID] vaccines are unlikely to completely sterilize a population. They are very likely to have an effect which works in a %, say 60 or 70%.'[182] Companies producing the COVID-19 vaccine are immune from liability diminishing their incentive to make them safe and regulators now have an amplified responsibility to monitor adverse events. 'Anything that happens to undermine the legitimacy of regulators to make independent decisions, is in my view, profoundly unhelpful,' said Sir John Bell in the abovementioned video. This highly-qualified scientist is also a member of SAGE (Scientific Advisory Group for Emergencies) and scientific advisor to the British government. He is part of the government's vaccine task force that has negotiated the purchase of vaccines to combat coronavirus.

Dr Michael Yeadon, ex-Pfizer head of respiratory research and Dr Wolfgang Wodarg, lung specialist and former head of the public health department, Flensburg, Germany, filed an application with the European Medicine Agency (EMA) on 1 December 2020 for the immediate suspension of all SARS-CoV-2 vaccine studies, in particular, the Pfizer/BioNTech study on BNT162b until safety concerns were addressed, especially that of female sterilization.

> 'The vaccine contains a **spike protein (see image) called syncythin-1**, vital for the formation of human placenta in women. If the vaccine works so that we form an immune response AGAINST the spike protein, we are also **training the female body to attack syncytin-1**, which could lead to infertility in women of an unspecified duration.'[183]

The information about Dr Yeadon and Dr Wodarg's claims was debunked by Bill Gates sponsored 'fact-checkers' as not true. It is 'not true' that Dr Michael Yeadon is currently the head of Pfizer Research as the article heading suggest, but a respected former vice-president and chief scientific officer of Pfizer.

Australia scraps billion-dollar coronavirus vaccine due to 'false positive' HIV

It was announced on 11 December 2020 that the Australian government has scrapped a coronavirus vaccine candidate being developed by the University of Queensland in partnership with the Australian global biotech company CSL after trial participants returned false-positive HIV test results. Prime Minister Scott Morrison said, 'the national security committee of cabinet agreed to terminate the purchasing agreement on Thursday, [10 December 2020] following expert health advice and fears the revelation would severely damage the Australian public's confidence in the COVID-19 vaccination program, which is expected to begin early next year.'[184] It's interesting how HIV false positives are not classified as HIV cases, whereas COVID-19 false positives are included as COVID cases. But why is HIV even being used in a vaccine to treat COVID-19?

Why Phase III clinical trials matter

A vaccine trial is a clinical trial to establish the safety and efficacy of a vaccine before it's licenced for general use. Clinical vaccine development is a multi-phase process.

Preclinical: The vaccine is tested in animals to see if it produces antibodies and protects against illness

Phase I: Small groups of people volunteer to trial the vaccine to make sure it is safe

Phase II: The clinical study is expanded and the vaccine is given to people in different demographic groups, e.g., age, physical health, similar to those for whom the new vaccine is intended, to see if it works

Phase III: Thousands of people are recruited and the vaccine is given to them to test for safety and efficacy

Phase IV: After the vaccine has been rolled out, ongoing surveillance is carried out to ensure the vaccine doesn't have any long-term adverse effects

Will vaccinations guarantee freedom?

Powerful voices tell us that life will never be the same; humanity will not be safe again until we are all vaccinated against this disease. Vaccines, we are told, are the answer and key that will unlock our personal freedom to work, travel and engage in community. Some people have embraced this notion wholeheartedly and are urging politicians and medical authorities to do everything in their power to accelerate this process. Others are more wary, knowing that a safe and effective coronavirus vaccine has never been produced thus far, and may never eventuate.

Scientists around the world were involved in a race against time to be the first to produce an effective vaccine which, according to reports, will be widely available in 2021. Normally, vaccine safety protocols are measured in years, not months, but steps in this process have been abandoned in the interests of urgency. The Bill and Melinda Gates Foundation is sponsoring vaccine research, manufacture and distribution in many countries worldwide.[185]

Dr Judy Mikovits, PhD, is not confident that a vaccine solution for COVID-19 will ever be found, commenting in the video *Plandemic* previously referred to, 'There is no vaccine currently on the schedule that works for any RNA virus.' Despite this, vaccine advocates in positions of power with incredible wealth are pushing their message relentlessly and that is to vaccinate everyone on Planet Earth. 'For the world at large, normalcy only returns when we largely vaccinate the entire global population,' said Bill Gates, billionaire co-founder of Microsoft and zealous vaccine advocate in the YouTube video 'Bill Gates–Normalcy only returns after global vaccination'.[186]

Conflict of interest

Half the patent for the Moderna/NIH vaccine is owned by the NIH and four NIH scientists have filed their own provisional patent applications as co-inventors.[187] Dr Mikovits is critical of this conflict of interests, commenting in the *Cairns News* article:

'It is a conflict of interest and in fact, this is one of the things I have been saying and would like to say to President Trump: Repeal the *Bayh-Dole Act*. That Act gave government workers the right to patent their discoveries. To claim intellectual property for discoveries that the taxpayer paid for. Ever since that happened in the early '80s, it destroyed science and this allowed the development of those conflicts of interests and this is the crime behind letting somebody, like Bill Gates with billions of dollars—nobody elected him—he has no medical background, he has no expertise, but we let people like that have a voice in this country, while we destroy the lives of millions of people.'[188]

Bill Gates has no medical training but he is a large sponsor of WHO and worldwide vaccine research and development. Dr Anthony Fauci, director of the American NIAID and once prominent member of the White House Coronavirus Task Force under the Trump administration, owns patents in many vaccines despite this research having been paid by the taxpayer, said Dr Judy Mikovits in her video *Plandemic*. It's incredible to think that people who are giving global advice for health either have no medical training and/ or own patents in the solution. One would naturally think this would be a grave conflict of interest, or one could believe that these gentlemen of means have honourable intentions!

Questions need to be answered, such as has there ever been a vaccine produced that is safe and effective against coronaviruses similar to COVID-19? The answer is no. 'Any previous attempts to produce an effective vaccine such as for the SARS viral outbreak in 2003 have failed, killing many people who were vaccinated,' said Dr Judy Mikovits. 'I can't even imagine the damage you can do with the vaccines currently being tested [for COVID-19],' she commented in her documentary video *Plandemic*. Judy Mikovits has maintained integrity in all she's done and stood for and has refused to bend to political coercion.

The flu vaccine as 'protection' for COVID-19

People have been strongly urged to get the flu shot as some protection amid the COVID-19 pandemic. The flu vaccine is between 40% and 60% effective against seasonal flu, according to a CDC article.[189] But Dr Judy Mikovits said it increases your risk of getting COVID-19 because of the contaminating gammaretrovirus strains injected with the flu vaccine.

According to Judy Mikovits, 'There is a lot of data to support COVID-19 is not SARS-CoV-2 alone, but that it is SARS-CoV-2 and XMRVs, HGRVs and including human gammaretroviruses and HIVs, and those are the people that are dying … People are dying from the combined symptoms that these viruses cause, such the deadly effect of the cytokine storm when the immune system goes rogue attacking and killing everything in sight including healthy cells in the body.'[190]

Supercharged fluad quad for older people

The supercharged flu vaccine recommended for people over

65 has four viral strains, including the H1N1 virus. The virus H1N1 was rampant in the swine flu epidemic of 2009, claiming many lives, and also the Spanish Flu of 1918–1919. This super-shot was administered to people in Italy where there is a large elderly population. It's this cohort in Italy that was devastated with COVID-19 in the early stages of the pandemic.

The Children's Health Defense Team, which includes Robert F Kennedy, Jr as board chairman, nephew of former American president John F Kennedy, said, 'Other studies have likewise pointed to increased risks of viral respiratory infections—both influenza and non-influenza—from flu shots. Shouldn't researchers be taking vaccination history into account when examining the staggering number of COVID-19 deaths that have occurred in nursing home residents subjected to annual influenza and pneumococcal vaccine requirements?'[191]

Despite all the rigorous media censorship contradicting the populist belief that vaccines, widespread repeated testing and contact tracing are our only answer, the alternative view is still getting out there for people who are prepared to stop, look, listen and learn.

Whistleblowers voicing their concerns

Highly-trained doctors in the field of microbiology, immunology and virology are voicing their concerns about the mainstream agenda purported to be engineered for a Big Pharma payday through email newsletters and newly-established private social media platforms such as www.brighteon.com, www.bitchute.com and https://questioningcovid.com. These brave doctors and other health advocates include Dr Sherri Tenpenny, Dr Judy Mikovits, PhD, David Brownstein, MD, Joseph Mercola, MD, Kelly Brogan, MD, Ben Lynch, MD, Dan Erickson, MD, Ty and Charlene Bollinger, Mike Adams and many others who have been instrumental in showing us the 'other side' workings of the scientific establishment with its criminal cartel of extreme corruption where lockdowns are being weaponised and innocent victims are being corralled into a vaccine holocaust.

The dark side of vaccines

An article appeared in *The Associated Press* highlighting how more polio cases are now caused by the vaccine than the wild type. 'Four African countries have reported new cases of polio linked to the oral vaccine, as global health numbers show there are now more children being paralysed by viruses originating in vaccines than in the wild.'[192] The Diphtheria-Tetanus-Pertussis (DTP) vaccine was discontinued in the USA and other western nations in the 1990s following thousands of child deaths and, as a consequence, the US switched from using whole cell pertussis to solely using acellular pertussis vaccines.[193] An acellular vaccine is a vaccine that may contain cellular material but does not contain complete cells.

Robert F Kennedy Jr. said, 'Girls vaccinated with the DTP vaccine—the flagship of Bill Gates's GAVI/WHO African vaccine program—died at 10 times the rate of unvaccinated kids.'[194] He was referring to a paper published by *The Lancet* where the researchers conclude, 'DTP was associated with increased mortality; OPV [oral polio vaccine] may modify the effect of DTP.'[195]

So, we have the DTP vaccine killing girls at 10 times the rate of unvaccinated kids and more polio cases now being caused by the oral polio vaccine than by the wild virus … and we should believe that combining the two will save lives!

Clinical study to find ways to coerce and manipulate people

There has even been a clinical study on finding the best ways to coerce and manipulate the general public—convince people to get the vaccine once it becomes available. The intention is based on social judgement; to shame people who decline the vaccine from a variety of angles including trustworthiness, selfishness, likeableness and competence to make personal decisions.[196]

There is a school of research within public health on how to frighten people, known as the 'fear appeal'. This is based on the premise that to successfully implement a public health measure, such as global vaccinations, you must first highlight a threat and that threat must be made personal. COVID-19 provided the threat. Enforcing lockdowns, mask-wearing, closing businesses and keeping children home from school has reinforced the fear, as will potential future directives that all people must be vaccinated and digitally tracked before they can resume a normal life.

Confusion takes an individual from fear to anxiety and when these elements reach a certain point, desperation sets in, at which time people are willing to do just about anything to get relief.[197]

The tactic of fear

In an interview between Molecular Interventions and Dr

Anthony Fauci in 2002, Dr Fauci talks about the climate of fear, like a double-edged weapon, and how a biological agent and terrorism are brought together as ingredients to create chaos. In that interview, Dr Fauci said, 'You know, bioterrorism is two things: It's a biological impact, and the terror that results from it. The disruption that Anthrax brought to our society was enormous compared to what the biological damage was: 18 people infected and five dead. That's unfortunate, obviously, and tragic for the people who died, but just look at the effects: It shut down the postal system, it shut down the Senate. It cost hundreds of millions, if not billions, of dollars in expenses for clean-up. It was a major disruptor.'[198] Create the problem, the reaction is predictable and the solution is in their favour! Connect the dots … it was Dr Fauci's SARS-CoV-2 gain-of-function research that was banned in the USA and he moved it to the Wuhan biosecurity lab in China.

If we believe the mainstream narrative and trust that our politicians, government authorities and Dr Fauci, Bill Gates, etc, have our best interests at heart, we will comply with dictated orders even if it means sacrificing our freedoms and liberties in the interests of the greater good. If we believe another, more sinister schema is at play, we can render psychological operations ineffective by seeing through the presented reality to the darker agenda beneath—the story behind the story. The future is in our hands. It's up to us what we wish to believe and what we think is incredible.

The purpose of this pandemic, or plague of corruption, is to make people fearful because, as we have seen, fear creates cooperation and control. The reason for this 'fearful' pandemic, some people say, is for an authoritarian takeover of our liberal democracy and to control the world population with mandated vaccines containing unknown substances which will kill many people in a form of eugenics while those remaining will be tagged via nanotechnology, such as with the injectable hydrogel biosensor for monitoring and surveillance to detect disease outbreaks in the community and modifying human behaviour through AI. This is discussed further in chapter six.

Money, power and control are huge motivating factors. Bill Gates, a major sponsor of WHO, is a proponent of population control and a genius with technology, while his friend and business associate, Dr Anthony Fauci, and his minions are using fraudulent science and revenue from vaccine patents to feed a narcissistic appetite for personal wealth 'while killing or maiming tens of thousands of people with contaminated vaccines or treatments that don't work', according to Dr Judy Mikovits. Dr Mikovits was originally employed by Dr Fauci in 1980 as a postdoctoral scholar in Molecular Virology at the American NIH National Cancer Institute and she has seen, first-hand, the corruption that takes place.

It's heartening to learn that more and more people worldwide are seeing through this perverse schema, which has had devastating financial and personal consequences, and realising there is an alternative agenda more sinister than most of us imagined possible. For many people, it's being likened to World War III but deploying biological instead of physical weapons. Knowledge, however, is power and, when equipped with such, we are better able to defend ourselves against a common enemy. Knowledge is our spring of hope, our ray of sunshine in the dark world of winter in which we currently reside.

A high volume of COVID-19 vaccine 'adverse drug reactions' expected

The United Kingdom's Medicines and Healthcare Products Regulatory Agency (MHRA) has sought an Artificial Intelligence (AI) system to process the expected high number of COVID-19 vaccine Adverse Drug Reactions (ADRs) by way of an urgent tender notice in a European Union public procurement journal, *Tenders Electronic Daily*, dedicated to European public procurement.[199]

In their bid for this contract, the MHRA highlighted the extreme urgency of this matter saying by way of explanation in the above tender, 'If the MHRA does not implement the AI tool, it will be unable to process these ADRs effectively. This will hinder its ability to rapidly identify potential safety issues with the COVID-19 vaccine and represents a direct threat to patient life and public health.'

'Direct threat to patient life and public health' is a disturbing claim from the MHRA despite the population being told that early trials support these vaccines as being safe and up to 95% effective. If safety and effectiveness are not an issue, why is the MHRA citing 'reasons of extreme urgency' in their bid to obtain a vaccine-specific AI tool to monitor the ADRs of a fast-tracked vaccine rollout? Under Regulation 32(2)c, as stated in the article 'Supplies - 506291-2020' *Ted - tenders electronic daily*, the MHRA claims that the expected flood of COVID-19 vaccine adverse reactions will overburden its current 'legacy system'. If the MHRA is aware that COVID-19 vaccines are potentially going to have a 'direct threat to patient life and public health', why aren't they reporting this information publicly? Why do we even need a vaccine when the large majority of COVID-19 cases are mild?

In the book *Corona False Alarm? Facts and Figures* by German doctors Karina Reiss and Sucharit Bhakdi,[200] the authors state that there have been 'fundamental flaws in data acquisition and especially on medically incorrect definitions laid down by the WHO', leading to the high number of COVID-19 cases. There have also been breaches in the rules of infectiology and reporting that 'violated all international medical guidelines' such as 'the absurdity of giving COVID-19 as the cause of death in a patient who dies of cancer'.

The CDC is now combining COVID-19 deaths with pneumonia and flu under a new category PIC (pneumonia, influenza and COVID). On the CDC COVIDView webpage, December 28, 2020, and updated weekly with US COVID activity, it states the 'levels of SARS-CoV-2 circulation and associated illnesses [pneumonia and influenza] declined or remained stable during the week ending December 19, 2020 [while] the percentage of deaths due to pneumonia, flu and COVID (PIC) has been increasing since early October.'[201] They are even using PIC, under the heading 'Mortality Surveillance' to state that cases are above the epidemic threshold. Of particular interest on this webpage under the heading '2020-21 Influenza Season Week 51 ending Dec 19, 2020' is a map of the US clearly showing minimal influenza activity for week 51, but for the prior season, 2019–2020 at week 51, it shows a completely different story.

Should vaccination be mandatory?

People who like to think independently may be well-advised to do their own research and make their own informed decision before submitting to vaccination.

Professor Jonathan Heeney, head of the Laboratory of Viral Zoonotics at the University of Cambridge and one of the people working on a vaccine, said that coronaviruses present a particular challenge to vaccine developers. He commented:

'If you make antibodies against the spike, they can end up binding to it and helping the virus invade important immune cells known as monocyte-macrophages. Rather than destroying the virus, these cells can then end up being reprogrammed by the virus, exacerbating the immune response and making the disease much, much worse than it would otherwise be.'[202]

The spike proteins are a primary focus for many COVID-19 vaccines being developed, including in Australia, as discussed in a report provided to Greg Hunt, MP, Minister for Health, from Dr Alan Finkel, Australia's Chief Scientist.[203] In this report, Dr Finkel says:

'Like other coronaviruses, SARS-CoV-2 has club-like spike proteins protruding from its surface. These spike proteins are essential for SARS-CoV-2 to bind to the host cell's 'ACE2' receptor, and once bound, the virus can then infect the host cell, replicate and infect more cells. These spike proteins elicit a strong neutralising antibody immune response, and are the primary focus for a majority of COVID-19 vaccines being developed.'

Vaccine immunotherapy—but a healthy immune system is paramount

Dr Mikovits said vaccines can be used as immunotherapy if they are manufactured safely under strict protocols and used with integrity. Nurturing the immune system by paying attention to a healthy diet and good nutrition, is paramount in not only protecting against disease but lessening the severity of symptoms if one is unfortunate enough to experience adverse consequences of this disease. Scientifically proven all-natural therapies offer hope for prevention, treatment and cure of many conditions and diseases, and this will be discussed in the next chapter.

Key concepts

- COVID-19 vaccines are now available but they are not a 'silver bullet' and their effectiveness is questionable. Hospitalised patients with severe infections are treated with remdesivir, dexamethasone and mechanical ventilation if indicated.
- There has been a lot of political controversy over the use hydroxychloroquine, an anti-malaria drug developed in 1946, and its precursor, chloroquine, developed in 1934
- Hydroxychloroquine has proven to be effective when combined with zinc and the antibiotic azotomycin in the early stages of disease. This protocol will end the COVID-19 plague, said Dr Vladimir Zelenko.
- Chloroquine, a drug related to hydroxychloroquine, was proved to act as a potent inhibitor of SARS coronavirus infection and spread in 2005, with the findings published in the *Virology Journal*
- A COVID-19 vaccine is not likely to guarantee freedom and may pose a direct threat to patient life and public health, including the risk of sterilisation

Pearl of wisdom

'It is not the strongest of the species that survives, nor the most intelligent. It is the one that is most adaptable to change.'

—Charles Darwin

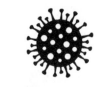

CHAPTER 4

Alternative Treatment

It was the spring of hope, it was the winter of despair

My story

My journey into thinking holistically began about 20 years ago when I injured my already wonky back doing goodness knows what. I was in excruciating pain and there came a time when I could only walk about six steps at a time and I had to sit down.

The local doctor and chiropractor could not do anything for me other than prescribe non-steroid anti-inflammatory drugs (NSAIDs), which did offer some relief. I was referred to an orthopaedic surgeon in Sydney, hoping that he would have some magic trick up his sleeve that would fix me instantly. There is nothing like instant gratification when you need it most! But I was not to be graced with such a quick remedy.

I explained my physical dilemma to this distinguished-looking specialist, adding that I didn't want to take anti-inflammatory drugs long-term as I was aware that they can cause stomach ulcers, and I didn't need any additional problems. After studying my medical history and x-rays, he told me, in a fairly brusque tone, that he couldn't do anything for me; that I would have to stay on NSAIDs for the rest of my life and that I would probably end up in a wheelchair.

That rather dire prognosis didn't sit comfortably with me, especially when I still considered myself quite young. There has to be another way, I thought, so I wended my way home with my husband and embarked on a long process of contemplative meditation. Thus, began my journey into nutritional medicine, and I haven't looked back.

My underlying spinal condition, described as 'moderately severe scoliosis', was diagnosed when I was a young teenager but it didn't cause me too many problems until later in years at a time when body maintenance becomes more challenging due to natural wear and tear. Conventional medicine couldn't offer me any hope other than physiotherapy and pain relief drugs and surgery was not recommended for my particular condition. Chiropractic, acupuncture and therapeutic massage became my main go-to therapies and, together with nutritional support, this has served me well for many years.

As you may have gathered by now, I am someone who likes to find an underlying cause for disease, and this calls for a lot of introspection. My type of scoliosis is described as idiopathic, or of 'unknown cause'. However, after much research, I believe it was caused, or at least contributed to by polio vaccines I had during my childhood of the 1950s and '60s. This conclusion was reinforced when I read the *Pub.Med.gov* journal article, 'Experimental scoliosis in primates: a neurological cause', where it states, 'Although a variety of techniques have been used with varying success to induce scoliosis in animals, primates have rarely been used. A series of monkeys is presented where scoliosis developed incidentally during the routine virulence testing of live, attenuated, oral poliomyelitis vaccines.'

Many polio vaccines in the 1950s and '60s were contaminated with the SV40 monkey virus. In the *National Institutes of Health* journal article, 'Patterns of polyomavirus SV40 infections and associated cancers in humans: a model', it advises, 'Potentially contaminated polio vaccines were used mainly from 1954 to 1963. Vaccines were supposed to be free from SV40 after mid-1961, but previous lots of vaccine were allowed to be used until stores were exhausted.'

So, if readers are wondering why I may favour non-conventional therapies to treat illness and disease wherever possible, now you know. Obviously, I have no proof, just a strong gut feeling of what may have caused my medical condition. I am not blaming anyone; this is what life has served up to me and the lessons I need to learn from it. Holistic therapies are my choice, and other people should be free to make their own choices, whatever they may be.

The immune system and how it works

True health can only be achieved by maintaining a properly functioning immune system. The immune system is complex and is constantly at work protecting the human body against bacteria, viruses, fungi, parasites and toxins. The cells of the immune system remain as individual cells, rather than forming into organs, and are present throughout the body. It's one of the most crucial systems in the human body and plays an essential role in human survival. To function properly, the immune system must detect a wide variety of invading pathogens and distinguish them from the body's tissue for destruction and elimination.

There are two main components of the immune system:

1. The innate or natural immune system which people are born with. It's always on alert and is the body's first responder against any foreign invader.
2. The adaptive or acquired immune system which kicks in after a week or two if the innate immune system has not been able to deal with the pathogenic invader. Its job is to fight a specific infection.

The innate immune system goes on the attack as soon as it recognises a pathogen as a foreign invader. It does this by identifying certain chemicals in the pathogen that tells the innate immune system they shouldn't be there. One example is white blood cells being recruited from the skin, mucous membranes, blood and body fluids by the innate immune system to fight bacterial infections causing redness and swelling when we have a cut.

The adaptive immune system has to learn the behaviours of a foreign invader and then produces 'helper cells' called T-lymphocytes and B-lymphocytes. T-lymphocytes are a type of white blood cell that reside in bone marrow and work to recognise things that can cause infection. When they bind with infectious cells, the T cells grow and divide quickly and overcome the invader.

While the T-lymphocytes are busy fighting off the invader, the B-lymphocytes are working to make antibodies to the infection. When these antibodies have been produced, the immune system will recognise the invader in present and subsequent infections and defend the body against it.

How the immune system is weakened

The immune system can become weakened due to poor dietary and lifestyle factors such as smoking, drinking alcohol in excess, poor diet and nutrition and lack of exercise and relaxation. Chronic diseases such as type 2 diabetes, cancer and HIV/AIDS can leave people immune-compromised, as well as medications and treatment such as corticosteroids and chemotherapy.

Some autoimmune diseases, where the body attacks normal healthy tissue such as type 1 diabetes, lupus and rheumatoid arthritis, also weaken the immune system. Having an overactive immune system, where the immune system reacts to substances in the environment that are normally harmless, can weaken it. These normally harmless substances can be dust, mould, pollen and various foods causing asthma, eczema and various allergies.

Being overweight or obese can weaken the body's immune system and reduce its ability to fight off infections, according to scientists. Metabolic syndrome, insulin resistance and low-grade chronic inflammation, characteristic of obesity, 'are associated with an overall negative impact on chronic disease progression, immunity from infection, and vaccine efficacy'.[204]

People with a weak immune system have a higher risk of not only contracting COVID-19 but also of developing more severe symptoms after exposure to the SARS-CoV-2 virus.

How to strengthen your immune system

The immune system can be strengthened by addressing the factors that caused it to become weak, paying particular attention to diet, nutrition and lifestyle choices. A healthy immune system can defeat invading pathogens and we need all the tricks up our sleeve now to bolster our immune system and protect us from COVID-19 and other diseases. Harvard Medical School advises that the first line of defence for a strong and healthy immune system is to choose a healthy lifestyle. When protected from environmental assaults and supported by healthy-living strategies, every part of our bodies, including the immune system, functions much better.[205] These healthy-living strategies include:

- Don't smoke
- Eat a diet high in fruits and vegetables.
  A Mediterranean diet is highly recommended.
- Exercise regularly in whatever form you prefer—walking, swimming, cycling
- Maintain a healthy weight
- If you drink alcohol, only drink in moderation
- Get adequate sleep and rest
- Take steps to avoid infection, such as washing your hands frequently and cooking meats thoroughly
- Try to minimise stress through relaxation techniques such as meditation
- Increase strength and flexibility through yoga, tai chi or qi gong
- Attitude is altitude—change your thoughts, change your life
- Be kind, be thoughtful and be genuine, but most of all, be thankful for what you *do* have

Importance of the immune system

Why is the importance of our natural immune system not being promoted? A healthy diet and good nutrition, along with exercise, rest and relaxation are paramount in maintaining a healthy immune system, but this is rarely, if ever, promoted by mainstream medicine. Why? Because it's not profitable to do so. Educational facilities teaching medicine are heavily sponsored by pharmaceutical companies and doctors are taught to promote chemical solutions that can be patented for profit.

Health agencies in the USA and Australia seem to have little interest in helping their citizens support their immune system through appropriate nutrition, preferring to rely on drugs and vaccines to treat diseases such as COVID-19. The British, however, appear to be embracing a more sensible, holistic approach and have issued nutritional guidance and recommendations to safeguard their populations. Researchers in the UK have also been actively involved in studies identifying the efficacy of certain nutrients, particularly vitamin D and the role it plays in preventing and treating viral infections.

The British Frontline Immune Support Team was founded by crowdfunding to make available some of the best quality immune support supplements free of charge to all National Health Service (NHS) healthcare workers who choose to be part of this initiative during COVID-19. Thousands of NHS workers have signed up for this community-supported scheme and are receiving their free nutritional supplements to help protect them from the infections they are exposed to daily.

Diet and COVID-19

Having a healthy diet is likely the most important factor in maintaining a healthy body and immune system and protecting us against disease, including COVID-19. It has been established, and mentioned previously, that 90% of people admitted to hospitals with COVID-19 had other comorbidities, many of which are lifestyle diseases that can be either prevented or reversed with proper attention to diet and adequate nutrition, exercise, rest and relaxation.

A study was conducted during March 2020 on patients hospitalised in 99 counties in 14 states of the US to determine the prevalence of underlying conditions of people with COVID-19 with the following results, 'Hypertension was the most common comorbidity among the oldest patients, with a prevalence of 72%, followed by cardiovascular disease at 50.8% and obesity at 41%. In the two younger groups, obesity was the condition most often seen in COVID-19 patients, with a prevalence of 49% in 50-64-year-olds and 59% in those aged 18-49 years.'[206]

Diabesity is the medical term for diabetes associated with obesity and is the leading cause of modern chronic disease. It's a state of being very overweight or obese and having type 2 diabetes, or one of the conditions, such as insulin resistance, that precedes it. Diabesity has become an epidemic, particularly in the Western world, and can lead to other serious health issues such as heart disease, cancer, kidney failure, dementia, blindness, hypertension and digestive disorders.

Diabesity has become a major problem worldwide, especially in the more affluent countries. Professor Paul

Zimmet, PhD, from the International Diabetes Institute, Melbourne, Australia states:

'In the last few decades, the number of people with diabetes has more than doubled globally. The International Diabetes Federation, using data from my International Diabetes Institute in Australia, recently reported that the number of people with diabetes will escalate from the present 246 million to 380 million by 2025. Despite the warning signs, most governments have been slow to act. Tragically, diabetes is now a global epidemic with devastating humanitarian, social and economic consequences.'[207]

Governments may be slow to act on this issue, but we can take action ourselves and be responsible for our own health and well-being. We can't rely on other people or governments to do that for us; it's a matter of self-responsibility and knowing how to cook nutritious, wholesome food, even on a budget.

Eat Your Medicine: Nutrition Basics for Everyone

Dr Mark Hyman, the author of several books on nutrition, has an excellent resource called 'Nutrition Basics for Everyone', an extract from *The Blood Sugar Solution* for people with diabesity and can be downloaded online.[208]

Choose a Mediterranean-style diet

The Mediterranean diet is based on traditional foods that people in countries like Italy and Greece used to eat and is nutritious and healthy for the general population. Researchers found that people in Mediterranean countries were generally very healthy back in the 1960s with a low risk of lifestyle diseases. Several studies have shown that the

Mediterranean diet can promote weight loss and reduce the incidence of lifestyle diseases such as heart disease, stroke and type 2 diabetes. The 'Mediterranean Diet 101: A Meal Plan and Beginner's Guide'[209] includes the following:

The Basics
Eat: Vegetables, fruits, nuts, seeds, legumes, potatoes, whole grains, breads, herbs, spices, fish, seafood and extra virgin olive oil.
Eat in moderation: Poultry, eggs, cheese and yoghurt.
Eat only rarely: Red meat.
Don't eat: Sugar-sweetened beverages, added sugars, processed meat, refined grains, refined oils and other highly processed foods.

Avoid These Unhealthy Foods
Added sugar: Soda, candies, ice cream, table sugar and many others.
Refined grains: White bread, pasta made with refined wheat, etc.
Trans fats: Found in margarine and various processed foods.
Refined oils: Soybean oil, canola oil, cottonseed oil and others.
Processed meat: Processed sausages, hot dogs, etc.
Highly processed foods: Anything labelled 'low-fat' or 'diet', or which looks like it was made in a factory.

Nutritional supplements may be needed

While it's important to eat a nutrient-dense and healthy diet, much of our food today, grown with modern agricultural practices, is nutrient deficient, and nutritional supplements may be warranted. Malabsorption syndromes such as coeliac disease or any illness/disease causing damage to the intestine from infection, inflammation, trauma, surgery or prolonged use of antibiotics can cause malnutrition. Elderly people are also prone to being malnourished due to eating smaller meals and not being able to efficiently absorb nutrients from their food due to wear and tear on the digestive system over time and lack of digestive enzymes in their biological makeup.

It's been scientifically proven that some nutrients in therapeutic doses can prevent, cure and treat disease as promoted by orthomolecular medicine. Orthomolecular medicine is, 'A therapeutic approach designed to provide an optimum molecular environment for body functions, with particular reference to the optimal concentrations of substances normally present in the human body, whether formed endogenously or ingested', as defined by Linus Pauling, molecular biologist, in *The Free Dictionary*. Further information about orthomolecular medicine can be found at www.orthomolecular.org.

Scientifically proven all-natural anti-viral substances

While some people have faith in properly-researched and tested vaccines and other pharmacological treatments, others have put their hope in nature's 'farmacy'—the many scientifically-proven, all-natural substances that have shown efficacy in treating many serious illnesses, including viruses.

The nutritional supplements that have been rigorously tested and received the most attention for treating viral illnesses are vitamin C, vitamin D, magnesium, zinc and selenium. Other nutrients include quercetin, found in many foods such as apples, cherries and dark berries, and EGCG in green tea. Both quercetin and EGCG act as ionophores, they transport zinc into the cells, similar to the action of hydroxychloroquine but weaker in efficacy.[210]

Vitamin C

Vitamin C exerts anti-viral activity in the body by increasing the production of interferons, as discussed previously, and also cited in the *Immune Network* journal article.[211] Vitamin C also aids healing in the body by its natural production of hydrogen peroxide (H2O2) to kill pathogens and microbes. Healthy human cells are protected from the oxidising effects of H2O2 due to the presence of catalyse enzymes. 'Vitamin C has a patchy history as a cancer therapy, but researchers at the university of Iowa believe that is because it has often been used in a way that guarantees failure', as reported in a *Science Daily* article.[212]

Vitamin C, in high enough doses divided throughout the day, is one of the best treatments for viral infections, with thousands of studies proving it, yet the public is being told that it's useless whenever it's discussed in the mainstream media. 'Oral supplementation with vitamin C (doses over 3g) appears to be able to both prevent and treat respiratory and systemic infections.'[213]

Despite the efficacy of vitamin C in treating viral and other diseases, doctors discredit it, without investigation, saying that it is not part of their 'training or belief system'. The medical system has been hijacked by those pushing the corporate pharmaceutical model, especially where large profits can be realised from newly patented synthetic drugs and vaccines, irrespective of whether or not they produce any desired results. Natural substances can't be patented for profit.

Medical knowledge and wisdom using botanicals and non-patented natural substances have been utilised with varying degrees of success over the centuries and the Chinese and South Korean people are using a range of vitamins and botanicals to treat this virus. A Twitter post from Dutch State Mines (DSM), producers of vitamin C, dated 3 February 2020 stated, 'Yesterday, 50 tons of immunity-boosting Vitamin C was shipped from our DSM Jiangshan plant to the Province of Hubei, of which Wuhan is the capital city.'

Dr Thomas Levy, a cardiologist and orthomolecular specialist, has written widely about the merits of vitamin C in his book *Primal Panacea*, where he tells the whole story of this amazing nutrient with hundreds of references to some of the thousands of studies conducted over the years on this essential vitamin. Dr Levy says, 'Very few viral and bacterial infections, except when already very advanced with multi-organ failure present or imminent, will fail to respond to this approach. Instead, a complete cure can routinely be anticipated. Much of the reason for this is that there is nothing more critical in restoring and sustaining immune system strength and tissue integrity than vitamin C.'[214]

Animals and plants all need vitamin C but guinea pigs, monkeys and humans have lost the capability to produce it during the course of evolution. A typical 70 kg goat is capable of producing 13,000 milligrams of vitamin C on a daily basis, said Dr Levy in his book *Curing the Incurable: Vitamin C, Infectious Diseases and Toxins*, yet the recommended daily intake of vitamin C for adults in Australia, according to the National Health and Medical Research Council, is a paltry 45 milligrams per day.[215] This minimum dosage may prevent scurvy but it won't provide therapeutic benefits for maintaining a healthy immune system and preventing or treating deadly diseases.

Dr Levy said, 'Epidemiologically, there's no question—if the whole population just took one gram or two grams a day, I believe it would have enormous impact on the general public health and the incidents of infectious disease.'[216] Dr Levy recommends taking two to three grams of vitamin C three or four times a day to enhance the immune system during active viral infection. Dr Levy said in this article, 'I personally believe, from the research and literature, vitamin C is the primary agent that stimulates and maximises the potency of the immune system. So, I don't think it can be undersold.'

Side effects of very high doses of oral vitamin C are the possibility of diarrhoea and/or nausea which can be immediately mitigated by temporarily reducing the dose and slowly titrating upwards if necessary. Liposomal vitamin C is better tolerated and much higher doses are achievable, having a similar effect to intravenous vitamin C treatments. The only contraindication for high dose vitamin C treatment is if the patient has a very rare glucose-6-phosphate dehydrogenase (G6PD) genetic disorder that interferes with the ability of red blood cells to bring oxygen to bodily tissues, causing a variety of symptoms related to anaemia, such as weakness and fatigue. This genetic disorder is more common in males of African and Mediterranean descent and is 'due to decreased glutathione [and] vitamin C levels inside the cell, [and] increased calcium levels inside the cell,' said Dr Levy in the abovementioned article. This can be supported by supplemental glutathione and magnesium.

Dr Levy recommends being tested for the G6PD genetic disorder before submitting to very high doses of vitamin C.

Liposomal vitamin C, the most effective form, was extremely difficult to purchase in Australia and from overseas companies during the early stages of the pandemic because many people know of its efficacy in treating viral illnesses and were stocking up on supplies.

A New Zealand farmer recovers from swine flu with vitamin C

Alan Smith, a dairy farmer from New Zealand, was holidaying in Fiji in 2009 when he contracted swine flu, an H1N1 virus. When he returned home, he was hospitalised in intensive care and placed in an induced coma on life support. He had developed 'white-out' pneumonia and was on the verge of death.

After three weeks with no improvement, Alan's doctors asked the family for permission to turn off his life support machines and allow him to die. Alan's family refused and requested that he be given high dose intravenous (IV) vitamin C, a registered medicine in New Zealand. The hospital very reluctantly agreed, as this form of treatment was not part of their normal treatment protocol. Alan was given 50 grams of IV vitamin C–25 grams one evening and 25 grams the following morning, and his response was spectacular. The following day a CAT scan of his lungs showed improved air flow and a dramatic improvement in his condition. The doctors refused to believe that his improvement was related to the IV vitamin C treatment, but rather 'turning the patient into the prone position' and discontinued the vitamin C treatment.

Further battles ensued with different doctors and their obstinate refusal to administer this life-saving nutrient. The family sought legal intervention and IV vitamin C was resumed but at a much lower dose of one to two grams per day. Alan made a slow recovery and, when he was well enough to be taken off life support and drink fluids independently, the family gave him oral vitamin C at six grams per day in divided doses in the highly absorbable form of Lypo-Spheric vitamin C, from LivOn Labs.[217]

Dr Thomas Levy has treated thousands of patients with vitamin C and is impressed with how oral Lipo-Spheric vitamin C is equal to or better than higher doses of vitamin C administered intravenously.[218] The combination of vitamin C and essential phospholipids radically improved cellular bioavailability. Less than 20% of IV C gets into cells. But the Lypo-Spheric compound permits 90% of the C to get into cells. That's because cell walls are made of fats. Vitamin C is water soluble. The tiny particles of vitamin C, when coated with phospholipids, have easier access to human cells.

Quercetin

Quercetin is a flavonoid found in herbs such as cilantro and dill, vegetables and fruit such as onion, kale, cranberries, apples, cherries and dark berries and its anti-viral properties have been investigated in numerous studies.

Like vitamin C, quercetin has antioxidant, anti-inflammatory, antiviral, immunoprotective and immunomodulatory properties.[219] When administered with vitamin C, quercetin's antiviral capability is enhanced— vitamin C helps recycle oxidised quercetin.

It has been demonstrated that quercetin also acts as an ionophore, transporting zinc across cell membranes, similar but weaker in effect to the action of the controversial drug hydroxychloroquine. Zinc is the mineral that stops the virus from replicating. 'Dietary plant polyphenols such as the flavonoids quercetin (QCT) and epigallocatechin-gallate [found in green tea] act as antioxidants and as signalling molecules. Remarkably, the activities of numerous enzymes that are targeted by the polyphenols are dependent on zinc. We have previously shown that these polyphenols chelate zinc cations and hypothesised that these flavonoids might be also acting as **zinc ionophores, transporting zinc cations through the plasma membrane**' [emphasis added].[220]

Another benefit of quercetin is that it appears to have the ability to bind to the spike protein of SARS-CoV, inhibiting its ability to infect host cells. This is discussed in the *Journal of Virology*, where the authors state, 'Two small molecules, tetra-*O*-galloyl-_-D-glucose (TGG) and luteolin were identified, whose anti-SARS-CoV activities were confirmed by using a wild-type SARS-CoV infection system … quercetin, which is structurally related to luteolin, offers great promise as a potential drug in the clinical treatment of SARS.'[221]

Vitamin D

Vitamin D deficiency has been identified as a significant risk factor for COVID-19 infection and death, with an estimated one billion people worldwide, across all age groups, affected.[222] This deficiency is particularly common during the winter months when people spend more time indoors away from natural sunlight. During winter, vitamin D stores, for most people, are at their lowest due to the weak winter sun not being able to stimulate the body to produce enough vitamin D. That's why they call winter the 'flu season'.

Having a vitamin D level of at least 55 ng/mL (138 nmol/L) lowers the possibility of contracting COVID-19 by 47% compared with those with a blood level below 20 ng/mL (50 nmol/L).[223] The lower temperatures and the humidity of the colder months are factors that influence the greater viability of SARS-CoV-2 in the air and on surfaces. As countries head into autumn, it's the ideal time for people to check their vitamin D blood levels and, if below 40 ng/mL (100 nmol/L), to take action and raise it above this level for optimum protection against COVID-19. This protective effect also extends to people with comorbidities—it lowers your risk, as discussed in the abovementioned paper.

Elderly people and people of colour most at risk of vitamin D deficiency

The demographic most severely affected by vitamin D deficiency are the elderly and people of colour. They are also the most adversely affected by COVID-19 infection, often with fatal consequences.

Elderly people are usually confined indoors, not only in winter but often all year round. People with dark skin have a reduced capacity to absorb vitamin D from natural sunlight because the increased melanin pigmentation in their skin acts as a natural sunblock. A *Forbes* study in America has identified that 42% of all COVID-19 deaths occurred in nursing homes and assisted living facilities.[224] Given that these people are also most likely to be severely vitamin D deficient due to their lack of exposure to natural sunlight, is this high death rate amongst the elderly in nursing homes just a coincidence?

Indonesia emerged as a COVID-19 hot-spot in June, recording more than 1000 new infections each day during the last week [7–13 June 2020],[225] said reporter James Massola in *The Sydney Morning Herald*, 19 June 2020. Also, in this publication, he says, 'On Thursday, [Indonesia] recorded 1331 new infections from just 10,381 people tested—that's an infection rate of nearly 13 per cent.' This northern neighbour of Australia is the fourth most populous country in the world, home to 270 million people, and the national government is showing few signs of making the tough decisions needed to clamp down on the rapidly growing infection rates. A working paper released by a team of Indonesian researchers shows a significant association between COVID-19 deaths and vitamin D deficiency with 96% having low vitamin D levels.[226] 'When vitamin D levels fall below 30 ng.ml (moderate levels) [75 nmol/L] people were 12 times as likely to die—and when they were even lower, below 20 ng/ml [50 nmol/L] people were 19 times as likely to die.' A study conducted in Spain found that eight in 10 hospital patients with COVID-19 were vitamin D deficient.[227]

Vitamin D reference ranges

Osteoporosis Australia recommends, as a general guide, most people should have a vitamin D level between 50 nmol/L and 70 nmol/L.[228] This means that if someone has a blood serum vitamin D level of 75 nmol/L or less, they have a 12–19 times higher risk of death from COVID-19 infection.

Dr Joseph Mercola was conventionally trained as a medical doctor in Chicago, USA, and became an osteopathic physician advocating natural health. He recommends, 'To improve your immune function and lower your risk of viral infections, you'll want to raise your vitamin D to a level between 60 nanograms per milliliter (ng/mL) and 80 ng/mL by fall. In Europe [and Australia] the measurements you're looking for are 150 nanomoles per liter (nmol/L and 200 nmol/L.'[229] Dr Mercola recommends monitoring vitamin D levels through blood tests and, if deficient, supplementing with the required dose to bring levels up to an optimal level for infection protection.

UK public health recommendations

The United Kingdom has been actively encouraging its citizens to supplement with vitamin D. In response to a journal article published in the *Nutrition Bulletin*, Public Health England issued its advice on vitamin D, recommending that those on coronavirus lockdown (including children, pregnant and breastfeeding women, and older people) should consider taking a daily supplement containing vitamin D even during the summer months if they were not going outdoors often.[230] As stated in this article, many people in the UK have low serum vitamin D concentration with a high prevalence of 39% among adolescent girls 11–18 years.

Vitamin D is one of the most important nutrients to optimise for COVID-19 prevention and it's strongly recommended to take magnesium and vitamin K2 to optimise vitamin D supplementation. 'Taking magnesium and vitamin K2 can lower your oral vitamin D requirement by as much as 244%.'[231]

The authors of the report *Stealth Strategies to Stop COVID Cold* say that it's your vitamin D blood level that matters, not the dose. 'Typically, the studies that fail to show a benefit of vitamin D supplementation used a specific dose of vitamin D rather than adjusting the dose to achieve an optimal vitamin D blood level.'[232] Also commented in the abovementioned report, 'Most people need about 8,000 units of vitamin D per day to achieve a healthy level of over 40 ng/mL.'

Despite significant scientific data backing the use of vitamins C and D, and showing the biology of how these nutrients and therapies can prevent and/or treat COVID-19, discussions and evidence showing the benefits have been banned and censored by government authorities and people in power pushing for vaccines and other pharmaceutical drugs such as remdesivir.

Zinc

Zinc is a trace element essential for a multitude of biological processes and deficiency is common. WHO reports that the global prevalence of zinc deficiency is 31% and is ranked the fifth-leading risk factor in causing disease worldwide.[233]

Zinc supplementation, in excess of biological requirements, can cause toxic effects. It should be used with care and limited to individuals who are identified as being zinc deficient. Some medical conditions such as pyroluria cause a zinc and vitamin B6 deficiency. 'Pyroluria is a familial disorder which occurs with stress, where an above-average amount of a substance consisting of 'kryptopyrroles' circulate in the body. The substance is harmless in itself, but high levels of these pyrroles systemically bind with B6 and zinc, preventing the use of these essential nutrients in the brain and body.'[234] It is believed that up to 10% of the population may have this metabolic condition.[235]

Zinc is important in supporting a healthy immune system and clinical deficiency manifestations include 'increased susceptibility to infectious diseases caused by bacterial, viral and fungal pathogens'.[236]

It's interesting to note that the loss of smell and taste are reported symptoms of early COVID-19 infection. Loss of these sensory abilities is also related to a zinc deficiency as the immune system uses more of this mineral in the process of fighting infection. As mentioned previously, zinc is part of the successful hydroxychloroquine (HCQ) protocol to treat COVID-19 where HCQ acts as an ionophore helping to transport zinc through the fatty membrane surrounding cells. Chloroquine, similar to hydroxychloroquine, is also a zinc ionophore, as well as the weaker, but more readily available, substances such as quercetin and epigallocatechin gallate (EGCG).[237]

The human body is a complex organism made up of trillions of cells, each with their own structure and function. Nutrients in peripheral blood are transported through the cellular membranes where healing takes place. Once inside the cells, zinc can help to inhibit a key enzyme involved in the replication of coronaviruses as indicated above and also by the authors of a review article published in *Biological Trace Elements Research* which says, 'The effectiveness of Zn can be enhanced by using chloroquine as an ionophore while Zn inside the infected cell can stop SARS-CoV-2 replication.'[238] Hydroxychloroquine is similar to chloroquine in its efficacy.

'A Novel Approach to Treating COVID-19 Using Nutritional and Oxidative Therapies'

Dr David Brownstein, et al, have been successful in treating patients diagnosed with COVID-19 with nutritional and oxidative therapies with 100% success. A small study consisted of 107 patients diagnosed with COVID-19, two of whom were hospitalised before commencing treatment and one who was hospitalised while receiving treatment. The conclusion of this clinical and translational research is as follows:

> 'In summary, we treated 107 COVID-19 patients, solely with biological therapies, who all recovered. Only three were hospitalised. Of the three hospitalisations, two were hospitalised before beginning our treatment and sought our care post hospitalisation. One was hospitalised while solely taking the oral regime of Vitamins A, C, D and iodine, and not the oxidative therapies. All recovered uneventfully. There were no deaths …
>
> As of this publication, no cure, treatment or preventative for SARS-CoV-2 has yet been proven effective in a randomized study, except for dexamethasone (a potent steroid) used in severely ill, hospitalised patients. In this study a novel treatment program, which is hypothesized to aid and support the immune system, was highly effective in the recovery of 100% of 107 patients. This case review points out that specific and relatively inexpensive nutritional support along with oxidative intravenous as well as intramuscular, and nebulized oxidative solutions may be helpful for COVID-19 patients.'[239]

MATH+ protocol

Five critical care physicians in the USA are having

great success treating COVID-19 patients with the MATH+ protocol they designed themselves, as discussed in the article 'Front Line Covid-19 Critical Care Alliance'.[240] COVID-19, in advanced stages, triggers hyperinflammation, hypercoagulation and hypoxia. Intravenous methylprednisolone, high-dose intravenous ascorbic acid, plus thiamine, zinc and vitamin D with full-dose low molecular weight heparin addresses these three core pathological processes. Oxygen support is also provided to avoid invasive mechanical ventilation.[241] The antiparasitic drug ivermectin is now being included in the MATH+ protocol.[242] This treatment is different from the standard care support and was largely ignored but is now receiving a more favourable response from the scientific community.[243]

Stop COVID Cold

A free downloadable report, 'Stealth Strategies to Stop COVID Cold', has extensive information on proven, natural, safe, effective and inexpensive ways to enhance your immune system and is available at www.stopcovidcold.com. There is also a two-minute COVID risk quiz to help people identify what their risk is for developing COVID-19 on this website.[244]

Seven steps to minimise your COVID risk

Under the 'Minimising Your Risk' tab on the www.stopcovidcold.com website, it identifies the following seven steps to minimise your COVID risk and they include:

1. Vitamin D is the key
3. Maximise your metabolic flexibility

4. Use quercetin with zinc

5. Monitor your omega-3 levels

6. Stay home if you have symptoms and sanitise often

7. MATH+ protocol if you get sick

8. More oxygen, fewer ventilators

Additional treatments available through orthomolecular medicine

Dr Thomas E Levy, MD, JD, is a cardiologist, attorney and author of a number of books including *Curing the Incurable: Vitamin C, Infectious Diseases, and Toxins*, *Primal Panacea* and *Stop America's #1 Killer*. He has written an extensive article, 'COVID-19: How can I cure thee? Let me count the ways', in which he lists many scientifically-validated natural therapies claimed to prevent, improve or cure this disease.[245]

Many of these therapies, such as vitamins C and D and the mineral zinc, have been discussed previously in this volume but there is merit in re-visiting these treatment strategies through Dr Levy's website, http://www.orthomolecular. org/resources/omns/v16n37.shtml due to their valuable contribution to health and wellness. Many other less-known therapies such as magnesium chloride, ozone and convalescent plasma, together with the previously-discussed treatments of hydroxychloroquine and chloroquine are also included in this very informative article referenced with links to scientific literature.

Dr Levy comments in this article, 'Many doctors get attacked for promoting treatments as cures for afflictions that are traditionally considered to be incurable. Certainly, some treatments promoted as being reliable cures are indeed either fraudulent or of only nominal benefit. However, failing to assert the validity of a true cure for a medical condition is just as detrimental to the health of an ailing patient as it is promoting a false cure.' He further states, 'While the politics of the COVID-19 pandemic are beyond the scope and aim of this article, there remain *no* valid medical reasons for not using any of the agents or interventions itemized above for either preventing or treating COVID-19 patients.'

Herd immunity

Herd immunity, in relation to contagious diseases, is a state when a population is immune from contracting the contagion either through vaccination or an immunity developed through previous infection. When a large percentage of a population becomes immune to a disease, the spread of that disease slows down or stops.

In some diseases, herd immunity can be triggered when 40% of the population becomes immune, but in most cases, this percentage is considerably higher. 'Once the level of immunity passes a certain threshold, the epidemic will start to die out because there aren't enough new people to infect,' said Natalie Dean from the University of Florida.[246]

Many factors affect herd immunity such as vaccination and previous exposure, mentioned above, but health status and a reduced fear response play a major role in protecting an individual from getting the disease in the first instance, due to the impact on the immune system.

In our current society, with the biomedical model of medicine, little attention is paid to natural immunity, as in the robustness of an individual's immune system.

Many people in our society are plagued with chronic diseases which are symptomatically managed under our current medical paradigm, but this does little to promote a strong immune system. Approximately 90% of patients hospitalised with COVID-19 have one or more underlying conditions, the most common being obesity, hypertension, chronic lung disease, diabetes and cardiovascular disease, as indicated in a CDC Morbidity and Mortality Report.[247]

When the majority of people in a group have been exposed to a microbe and have developed immunity, it offers some protection to all people in that community, regardless of the presence of susceptible individuals, such as those with compromised immune systems and the elderly. If a majority of young people, who usually are not severely affected by COVID-19, contract the disease, recover and gain individual and, consequently, herd immunity, they 'protect' the susceptible people from contracting the disease because the virus has run out of easily accessible hosts to infect. Microbes can also mutate into less pathogenic strains and die a natural death. Alternatively, microbes can mutate into more virulent strains and hang around in the community for a longer period of time, causing a dilemma for vaccine researchers.

For a visual interpretation of how herd immunity was achieved historically in North America, Europe and the South Pacific during the outbreaks of measles, tuberculosis, survey, pertussis, scarlet fever, influenza and diphtheria, see 'Immunization Graphs: Natural Infectious Disease Declines: Immunization Effectiveness; and Immunization Dangers', prepared by Raymond Obomsawin, PhD.[248] Also see the vaccine effort in Australia in a historical perspective and how herd immunity was achieved.[249]

Herd immunity is a very tricky and controversial subject because there are so many variables involved and it depends on which epidemiologist you listen to for their interpretation of these variables. According to modelling, natural herd immunity can be acquired without vaccination when somewhere between 10% and 70% of a population become infected and recover. Researchers applying statistical modelling to the COVID-19 pandemic have generally taken divergent approaches to modelling, which, in turn, have yielded highly variable and inconsistent estimates.

Epidemiologists have suggested that herd immunity can be achieved when 60–70% of the population has been infected and recovered or vaccinated. Tom Britton, a dean of mathematics and physics at Stockholm University in Sweden, says that particular percentage assumptions are flawed. 'Exactly what the number is, we don't claim to know … Our particular model, rather than 60% [herd immunity], was 43%. But we don't claim 43% to be a magic number. I think the actual number is substantially lower than people actually believe.'[250] This would also depend on how effective the vaccine was. Dr Anthony Fauci, director of the NIAID, has warned that a vaccine, once approved, may only be 50% to 60% effective. Dr Fauci said in a webinar hosted by the Brown University, 'The chances of it [the vaccine] being 98% effective is not great which means you must never abandon the public health approach.'[251] Dr Fauci also said, 'The first coronavirus vaccine may not be the miracle cure we've been hoping for … A coronavirus vaccine that is only 50% effective would still be acceptable and liable to be given the green light by the Food and Drug Administration (FDA).'[252]

In the article 'Will the US achieve COVID-19 herd immunity before a vaccine?' Professor Gabriela Gomes, statistician at the University of Strathclyde in Glasgow, produced a model suggesting that herd immunity may be achieved when 10–20% of the population has been infected and recovered from this disease. She said that we may even be close to this now, especially in countries or cities that have been heavily impacted by this coronavirus. She further said, 'Traditional models often assume that everyone is susceptible to a virus based on the average susceptibility of the general population.' This has huge implications in relation to the general health and well-being of a population. Generally speaking, the healthier a person is, the less susceptible they will be to becoming infected with a disease such as COVID-19. A properly functioning immune system acts as a very effective defence against COVID-19 and any other disease, which is exactly what it was designed to do. Herd immunity is what we need to aim for as a positive outcome in any pandemic. Other positive and negative pandemic outcomes will be discussed in the next chapter.

Key concepts

- The importance of a healthy immune system in preventing disease
- Scientifically proven all-natural anti-viral nutrients—vitamins, minerals and other natural substances have been shown to inhibit coronavirus replication in the body
- Vitamin D deficiency is a significant risk factor for COVID-19 infection and one of the most important nutrients to optimise COVID-19 prevention

- Elderly people and people of colour are most at risk of vitamin D deficiency
- How hydroxychloroquine and zinc work together to treat COVID-19
- The MATH+ protocol success in treating COVID-19

Pearl of wisdom

'Good health is not something we can buy. However, it can be an extremely valuable savings account.'

—Anne Wilson Schaef

PART 3

The Solution: Building Hope and Resilience

CHAPTER 5

Positive and Negative Outcomes

It was the epoch of belief, it was the epoch of incredulity

No more laissez-faire

We thought we had it all before COVID-19—knowledge, wisdom and insight. Things in Australia were quite cosy, relatively speaking, compared with other countries. Business was booming, unemployment was low and the economy was bouncing along in fairly fine style. Wise decisions had laid solid foundations for the land of golden opportunity where the often laissez-faire lifestyle went hand-in-hand with, 'she'll be right mate, put another shrimp on the barbie.'

We lived with nature, adjusting and adapting to the hiccups of history—war, famine, drought, bushfires, floods, pestilence and disease. They all came with their challenges, but as stoical citizens, we rose to the occasion, supported each other and did what was necessary to recover. We learnt wisely from the experiences, adjusted our lifestyles and were comfortable with the outcomes. We thought we were wise, but on reflection, how foolish we were. According to Socrates, 'The only true wisdom is knowing that you know nothing.'

The enemy of by-gone days could be seen and heard with the physical senses, but we were not prepared for a devious monster sneaking through the air like a thief in the night. There was an undercurrent at play, a rip in the ocean of life, catching us unprepared, off-guard and dragging us into uncharted waters. Were we foolish to trust that all was fine and dandy with Planet Earth, our environment, scientific community and relationships with each other? Have we put too much trust in the scientific community, political leaders and the media? Deeper truths are often revealed in a time of crisis.

While it's heartening to see some silver linings in our new reality and some of our restrictions are being gradually eased, dark clouds still hang around like a menacing stalker, generating fear in the unwary. We will survive this form of biological terrorism and we will thrive, but it's going to take some serious and truthful soul searching to do so.

With courage and kindness, we will find our truth. One of Sir Winston Churchill's famous quotes is, 'Fear is a reaction; courage is a decision and it is the courage to continue that counts.' In a speech presented by Senator Marise Payne, 16 June 2020, she said, 'We must stand up for our values and bring our influence to bear in these institutions to protect and promote our national [and personal] interests.'[253]

Conflicting messages

The general public is very confused about everything relating to this pandemic, and this confusion is causing panic and fear. We have received so many mixed and contradictory messages that people are left very perplexed and don't know what to believe.

This confusion applies even to our own government-mandated orders, such as it was okay to ride on public transport with other people but it was not okay to go for a joy ride in your personal vehicle, your own private 'bubble', or fish alone from a boat in the middle of a lake. It was okay for essential workers to continue working, but it was not okay for those considered non-essential to earn a living unless they could work from home. It was okay for larger stores to remain open, but not smaller ones, which were forcibly closed. It was forbidden to walk on deserted beaches or for parents to take their children to empty playgrounds. Tattoo parlours were allowed to operate at a time when people were not allowed to attend church for worship. Limits were imposed on the distance travelled from our place of residence, interstate borders were closed, overseas travel banned and all mass gatherings were cancelled.

COVID-19 seems to be like a changing tide, ebbing and flowing at its unpredictable whim. As countries work to flatten the curve and ease their restrictions, outbreaks happen again, leading to more diagnosed cases and further restrictive measures. Some government and medical authorities argue that we should be aiming for the elimination of this virus by imposing very severe lockdown and social distancing measures, crippling an already severely damaged economy, while others say that elimination is not practical and that we should aim for suppression.

The Australian Government Chief Medical Officer, Dr Nick Coatsworth, said in an opinion piece, 'We have pursued aggressive suppression with the knowledge that this will lead to periods of elimination in parts of the country. Pursuing elimination and suppression are not mutually exclusive concepts; rather a continuum that can be adjusted to local circumstances.'[254]

Positive outcomes

Homelessness improves

A positive outcome to emerge from the COVID-19 pandemic is that many homeless people now have permanent accommodation. In New South Wales, 100 people have been placed in permanent accommodation during April and May 2020 compared with approximately 200 per year under normal conditions. These people now feel safe and no longer need to concern themselves with the insecurity of being homeless or having their belongings stolen.

Before the COVID-19 lockdown took effect, the Australian Government moved thousands of homeless people off the streets and into temporary accommodation in hotels, motels and student accommodation scattered around the major cities and in some country areas. It was an emergency measure, the scale of which Jenny Smith, chair of Homelessness Australia, had never seen before.

The coronavirus shutdowns had a knock-on effect of job losses and other domestic issues, forcing some people out of their homes onto the street to 'sleep rough' for the first time. This particularly applied to people who didn't qualify for the newly-established federal government JobKeeper allowance or other welfare support, such as casual employees who hadn't been employed in the one job continuously for 12 months or foreign nationals temporarily residing in Australia.

The majority of people sleeping rough have been doing so for many years and having no fixed address made it difficult for welfare agencies to offer and provide support. With this demographic now largely accommodated, at least temporarily, social workers have found they have a captive audience and can help them to deal with substance abuse and issues relating to mental health and childhood trauma— the primary causes for their unfortunate predicament. When a homeless person's self-esteem and domestic life improves, so does their job prospects and the likelihood of a return to worthwhile employment.

Homelessness is not inevitable. It can be fixed, according to advocates, as stated by The Australian Broadcasting Corporation news reporter Ben Knight. On a national scale, it costs the taxpayer approximately \$13,000 less each year per tenant to have homeless people accommodated. Bevan Warner, CEO of Launch Housing in Melbourne, said it costs much more than this amount in police callouts and having medical staff treat people in emergency wards.[255]

The question now remains whether approximately 7000 people are going to be turfed out of temporary accommodation and back on the streets when this pandemic ends. A potential solution to this problem could be converting some empty office space, made redundant by employees continuing to work at home, into permanent social housing.

Employees working from home

For many people, working from home has worked well and this trend is likely to continue. With the advent of technology, location for many areas of employment has become less relevant. People previously working in city-based businesses and living nearby, can now live in regional areas and successfully carry out their work requirements from home. This offers a more flexible and family-friendly environment for employees, especially those with young families, who can now more easily work around family priorities. Employers benefit by enhanced production with happier, less-stressed staff and a reduced requirement for expensive office accommodation.

For some people during the pandemic, working from home has meant they have been able to take their elderly parents out of nursing home care and care for them themselves in their own homes. Nursing homes have become hotspots for COVID-19 infections and people who can accommodate their elderly loved ones at home can now do so and feel relieved that their parent is less likely to become infected with this disease.

Business innovation

Many businesses have had to reinvent themselves to stay afloat in a rapidly changing world while trying to maintain a 'business as usual' philosophy. They've had to embrace a steep learning curve into the world of rapid digitalisation to offer services online. Some businesses changed their focus altogether to cater for emerging markets, such as distilleries around the world switching from spirits to hand sanitiser to cater for a global shortfall sparked by COVID-19.

Cleaner environment

Carbon emissions are down globally. The effect of fewer commutes by employees during the lockdown period has meant fewer vehicles on the roads and a cleaner environment. Air quality in big cities has improved considerably; Mount Everest was visible from more than 200 km away due to coronavirus lockdowns resulting in the cleanest air over Nepal in many years, and the reduction in deadly air pollution in China has saved many lives.

Return of manufacturing jobs

Other positives during the pandemic include the return of some manufacturing jobs in Australia, especially for basic medical supplies and other necessary commodities, to reduce our vulnerability when overseas supply chains are broken. Additional priority areas for self-sufficiency include the manufacture of steel for building projects and solar panels for our energy requirements.

'We have the capacity to attract the best brains in the world, we also have the capacity to lead the world in some areas like advanced manufacturing,' said New South Wales Premier Gladys Berejiklian in a *Financial Review* article.[256]

Automation and robotic technologies will largely replace people on the factory floor. Some jobs will disappear, but others will be created, offering opportunities for people to reskill into more secure industries. Gladys Berejiklian said that in a post-COVID-19 world, we will focus on manufacturing, healthcare and infrastructure. She also said that Australia could market itself as a COVID-19 safe location, ideal for investment and travel, particularly as we have managed to come through this pandemic so far (February 2021) with relatively few causalities compared with other countries.

Community support and connectedness

Another good thing to emerge from this pandemic is that it has brought some people closer together in the spirit of community support and comradeship. People out walking, with more time on their hands, are now stopping to chat, often with strangers. Other people have put their own lives in danger by volunteering to assist in public health high-risk areas, such as undertaking light administrative duties in medical settings, taking the pressure off doctors and nurses, and welcoming and screening visitors to aged care facilities. Gym instructors, entertainers and other businesspeople, recently unemployed due to lockdowns, have embraced technology to instruct and entertain via Zoom and similar online platforms at little or no charge, greatly benefiting the wider community.

People are finding new ways to stay connected. Some people have created music from their balconies, joining together with their voices and instruments to entertain everyone within listening distance. Street dance parties, maintaining social distance, have been held in some locations, adding a little joy to some people's lives and reinvigorating a sense of social cohesion.

Another good thing about this pandemic—a weird silver lining in this horrible atrocity—is that people have had time to think in lockdown. The pace of life has slowed and some businesses have ground to a halt or are working in slow motion. Housebound people are indulging in handicrafts and DIY projects, cooking up a storm and growing vegetables in droves. They are getting back to nature, tuning into their inner thought processes and re-assessing their values.

Education has become digitalised and affordable

While some students may struggle with learning from

home and miss the company of their classmates, it does come with some benefits. Educational institutions can now save on infrastructure costs and these savings can be passed on to the students, making education more affordable and accessible. Parents also get first-hand knowledge on how lessons are taught, can participate more fully in their children's education and have a greater understanding of how their child is progressing.

Extending kindness and generosity

A different but equally delightful experience for many was when a farmer near Greenethorpe, New South Wales, grew a crop of sunflowers alongside a public road purely to put a smile on the face of anyone who passed by. Travellers were also allowed access into the paddock to pick sunflowers and take them home; happy flowers to remind them of a happy time. This simple act of kindness and generosity on the farmer's part brought considerable cheer to many people, easing their stressful burdens, even if only temporarily.

Negative outcomes

Fear-based response

There is a lot of fear generated around this disease. Some people are calmly accepting the current situation, stoically taking it in their stride. They are doing what needs to be done with dutiful obligation believing this too, will pass. Others believe the worst, thinking we're all condemned if we don't surrender our freedoms and liberties and become prisoners of the state for our own protection.

Gone are the days of carefree lifestyles where we can choose to come and go as we please and socialise with family and friends ad libitum. Everything from eating and shopping to travel and engagement with community now has reservations with suspicion, stigma and social distance attached. The spontaneity of life is gone as people wonder and worry about catching COVID-19 from their family, friends and associates. People have become wary and cautious as the virus erodes not only our human friendships and interactions but also deprives us of time in nature as we shelter in place.

Since 11 March 2020, when COVID-19 was declared a pandemic, the world has been ordered into social distancing and varying degrees of lockdowns because it was predicted that people would be dying like flies with the remainder living in fear of being infected or infecting someone else. Fear triggers a paralysis in rational thinking and people succumbed to the dictates of authoritarian institutions and governments, believing that science and those in positions of power know best. We reluctantly surrendered our constitutional rights, such as the freedom of speech, assembly, privacy and the right to work for the greater good of public health.

Sometimes it's not the disease itself that kills people, but the fear of it. Fear creates stress, and stress wreaks havoc on the human body and all its intricate and interdependent systems. Sun Tzu said in *The Art of War*, 'If you know the enemy and know yourself, you need not fear the result of a hundred battles.' One of Nelson Mandela's powerful insights is equally poignant, 'Know your enemy—and learn about his favourite sport.' The more we know about what is really going on, especially behind the scenes, the better equipped we will be to protect ourselves and our loved ones, not only from the virus itself but also from the dictates of authoritarian power that may not have our best interests at heart.

Fear causes up to 90% of all disease

Dr Bruce Lipton, the author of *The Biology of Belief*, said in an article that fear generates stress in the human body, causing up to 90% of all disease. He encourages people to let go of fear. When we live with chronic fear consciousness, when it's with us all the time and not only in times of fight-or-flight emergency, it becomes ingrained in our consciousness and wreaks havoc on our immune system.[257]

Chronic fear releases stress hormones and changes our body chemistry. The adrenal system shunts blood flow and nutrients to where it is needed most in times of stress, such as the heart and lungs, at the expense of the immune system. Dr Bruce Lipton emphasises, 'We have to recognise that most of the fear is just programming; people scaring us with beliefs about this is going to happen and that's going to happen. And when we hold those beliefs in our mind, those beliefs are translated into the chemistry of stress, which then impacts the body in a very negative way.' Every time fear comes up, he suggests changing the story in your mind to something more pleasant because 'fear itself is the cause of the illness and the fear is the result of consciousness.'

Fear as a tool for manipulation

Fear is arguably one of the easiest ways to manipulate people but when people look at the facts logically and take the emotion out of the situation, they will see it for what it really is. We hear a lot about total case numbers, but we hear very little about people unaffected by the virus or those who have recovered. The media is focused on a scare campaign of fearmongering to make people complicit in begging for a vaccine rather than having it forced upon them, irrespective of any potentially deadly side-effects or changes to our DNA. As more and more people let go of fear and return to rational thinking, they are waking up to what's really happening, opening up public conversations about science, health and liberty despite major attempts by Big Pharma and Big Tech, working with governments and mainstream media to censor them.

Censorship is rife and this also generates fear as our freedom of speech, a basic human right, is being taken away from us in totalitarian style. If any conversation borders on questioning the orthodox narrative, it's immediately pounced on by the 'thought police' and either debunked or censored from all forms of media. The 'thought police' are treating citizens like imbeciles, unable to make everyday decisions and risk assessments themselves.

It's been an eye-opener to see just how many tentacles the censorship monster has, but the truth is still getting through, like a tenacious dog reluctant to give up a bone, before it is pounced on again and condemned. YouTube videos that don't favour Big Pharma, Big Tech and Big Business are a prime target. Free speech has been condemned, and this is contraindicated in the Universal Declaration of Human Rights, where it states clearly that 'human beings shall enjoy freedom of speech and belief and freedom from fear and want.'[258]

How to counteract fear

Apart from fear being used as a tool against people to manipulate them into compliance, it can also be used to empower people and free them from the chains of emotional bondage.

Fear has been used as a manipulative power since time immemorial to coerce people into doing something for another agenda. Buy and use this product and you will live longer, do this and we will save lives and livelihoods. Fear agendas are played out almost daily in political parties worldwide to gain supremacy and induce obedience. Facing fear gives us courage and, by failing to face it, we can become imprisoned in it, causing all kinds of grief and anxiety issues.

When people are afraid of something and bravely face up to it with knowledge, determination and appropriate action, the anxiety generated by fear will fall by the wayside and disappear into nothingness. We are only fearful of what we don't understand. When we understand more of what is going on in any given situation, we fear it less—ignorance is a prerequisite of fear. If we change the perception of how we see fear and understand the mechanisms generating it, we will realise that, in many cases, it is simply false evidence appearing real.

If anyone is experiencing fear in their lives and relationships due to COVID-19 or any other cause, it's recommended they seek appropriate assistance from a medical professional. In addition, people experiencing fear may find the Emotional Freedom Technique useful.

Strategies to reduce stress, fear and anxiety
- Limit your exposure to negative COVID-19 news
- Pay careful attention to loaded terms such as statistics, total cases, deaths and unstated assumptions
- Don't take everything you hear as gospel. Ask questions about what you are being told

- Pay attention to diet and nutrition—eat whole foods and limit sugar
- Get quality sleep
- Exercise regularly
- Practice mindfulness meditation
- Use the Emotional Freedom Technique (EFT)[259]

Emotional Freedom Technique

The Emotional Freedom Technique, developed by Gary Craig, was introduced to the public in 1995. It's a form of needleless acupuncture that can be practised by anyone anywhere. It uses the Chinese meridian system in a process of tapping on meridian points with the fingertips. This, together with identifying the 'problem' in the mind and repeating positive affirmations, realigns the disrupted meridian by balancing or unblocking the energy flow.

While primarily providing emotional health, it can also offer relief from various physical symptoms such as muscular pain and headaches.[260]

Mental health

The COVID-19 response has taken a huge toll on the mental health of citizens worldwide with symptoms of fear, stress, anxiety and depression. Students unable to return to classroom studies are afraid of being left behind by their peers and concerned about the impact this may have on their career prospects. Citizens are unable to return to their birth country to attend funerals of loved ones and be with extended family members at this point. Elderly residents in nursing homes are unable to have family and friends be with them in their hour of need, and often die alone.

From a psychological perspective, the loss of control and inability to plan and set goals is unsettling for many.

Emi Golding, psychologist and founder of the Workplace Mental Health Institute said on *ABC Radio* Saturday AM on 15 August 2020, 'When we don't have control over our life, we get this sense of helplessness. When we don't know how long that is going to last for, with all the uncertainty about when the restrictions are going to be lifted, then we get hopelessness. So, it is not just the family connections, it is also being able to plan and be in charge.'

The uncertainty for many people and potentially all people is that we don't know how long this virus is going to be with us. Potentially, it could be a plague on our landscape for years, if history is anything to go by. Or it could perhaps burn itself out over a short period, such as with the SARS outbreak in 2003, and become relatively insignificant.

If COVID-19 is with us for a longer term, it's important to understand that while we may be able to pull together in the short-term and tolerate lockdowns and social restrictions in the name of public health, we need to be able to put long-term strategies in place to reduce anxiety, uncertainty and tension. Emi Golding had the following suggestions on *ABC Radio* referred to above:

'At an individual level, it is about planning what we can. Regaining that sense of control by saying I may have had this list of objectives for 2020, or ideas on what I wanted to do this year, and now that looks like it is not going to be possible, at least not in the way I had originally planned. So how can I re-think this and still achieve what I want to do in a different way, or what else can I do instead, so I can still have this sense of progression, of moving forward with things.

Because we know that it is important for us as humans to have goals, to be able to move forward, so it is getting the right balance between being kind to yourself if you don't achieve everything that you wanted to do, but also moving forward where you can.'

Domestic violence

Our country has been forced into a recession, the economy has been decimated, many businesses are struggling or have closed permanently and unemployment continues to rise in many countries. This is despite unprecedented welfare strategies sponsored and enacted by many governments to mitigate these effects.

But the cost goes even deeper. The 'black dog' of depression has haunted many families, domestic violence has skyrocketed, along with suicides, and child abuse has reached an all-time high. Google reported a 75% surge in searches for domestic violence in the two months since the shutdown began in March 2020, and domestic violence crisis lines have experienced a 250% increase in referrals to after-hours services, according to an article published in *Marie Claire*.[261]

Many women in domestic violence situations are hesitant to leave believing 'the danger they know is safer than the danger they don't', according to Jacqueline Cunningham, the CEO of a Queensland-based service, Safe Haven Community, that helps place vulnerable women in safe accommodation when they have nowhere else to go. 'One of the most frightening aspects about the current crisis is not just the reported influx of women seeking help from domestic violence services, but the ominous silence from those who aren't,' she said, as reported in the abovementioned *Marie Claire* article.

Child abuse

Child abuse has increased dramatically since the commencement of COVID-19 lockdowns with police data indicating in *The Canberra Times* newspaper, 'Material shared on the dark web between February and March doubled from this time last year.'[262]

When children stay indoors, they often spend more time online, with some being groomed and then blackmailed to produce more and more extreme material, according to the abovementioned article. In other instances, adults with access to children are being groomed online to carry out these heinous crimes.

There is also an online grooming manual, a predator handbook 'describing ways to manipulate and exploit the increased number of children at home and online during COVID-19', Australia's eSafety Commissioner, Julie Inman Grant, said in *The Guardian*, Australian edition.[263] The handbook advises predators to get their kicks online, rather than trying to meet children face-to-face.

Research commissioned by the Australian Centre to Counter Child Exploitation indicated only 52% of parents and carers talked to children in their care about online safety, as reported in the abovementioned article. The Australian Federal Police advise that the best way to protect children is to be aware of the risks associated with spending time online and talking to them about their online activities.[264]

'The United Nations Population Fund has predicted that for every three months lockdowns continue, an additional 15 million cases of domestic violence will occur worldwide.'[265] Domestic and family violence and the associated mental health consequences are the unintended, potentially long-term consequences of COVID-19, an additional pandemic, which the media is not broadcasting and politicians are keeping very quiet about.

Suicide

There is a silent pandemic, greater in intensity, lurking in the shadows of COVID-19 and that is the increasing rate of suicide in Australia. No one is talking about it. It's a silent death toll and little is being done to drive the numbers down.

'The predicted increase of suicides is 25% each year for the next five years,' Professor Ian Hickie, co-director of the Brain and Mind Centre at The University of Sydney said in a news article.[266] 'That's 750 extra deaths by suicide a year [in Australia]. It's an enormous number. It will be a massively bigger death toll than COVID.' Professor Hickie also said that the predicted 25% more suicide deaths annually could end up being a conservative estimate. New modelling by Sydney's Brain and Mind Centre indicates 'a projected increase of up to 30% among young people aged 15-25 years'.[267]

The Australian Bureau of Statistics and other studies are showing an increased rate of psychological distress since the onset of the pandemic. Initially, there was a high degree of anxiety about health, but that anxiety is now more about economic implications for people at present and in the future. Mental health, on a broad scale, is being impacted due to uncertainty about the future, with disruption to lives and livelihoods causing increased pessimism as lockdowns become common and the situation becomes chronic.

The Australian Men's Health Forum (AMHF), a peak body for men's health in Australia, said that social isolation increases male suicide risk, particularly for older men, those who have lost their jobs and livelihoods, and men with fewer social connections, including fathers who have been separated from their children. Glen Poole, CEO of AMHF said, 'We support the Government's decisive action to save as many lives as we can from coronavirus and this needs to be balanced with innovative action to save more lives from suicides linked to isolation and financial distress in the coming months.'[268] Online support services include virtual Men's Sheds and other groups such as Dads in Distress and Mr Perfect are using Facebook and other social media platforms to keep men connected.

Long-term effects—health

It is difficult to determine, or even estimate, the accurate number of COVID-19 recoveries and long-term effects because many cases are so mild that they go unreported. Most people recover without any further incident and some people who recover quicker from COVID-19 continue to have antibodies against SARS-CoV-2 for several months.[269]

The long-term effects of this disease are more pronounced in the 20% of people who have moderate to severe symptoms, and particularly the five percent who require intensive care in hospital. The speed of recovery in this group and the development of lingering symptoms is not a linear process, Dale Needham, a critical care physician at Johns Hopkins School of Medicine said in a *The New York Times* article on 1 July 2020.[270] It's very individualised, according to the patient's general health at the onset of disease and any inherent weaknesses they have.

Dr Zijian Chen, medical director of the Centre for Post-COVID Care at Mount Sinai Health System, said in the abovementioned article that the biggest problem he was seeing at the centre in patients after leaving hospital was shortness of breath due to heart or lung impairments or a blood clotting problem. He also said that some patients have a lingering cough that makes it hard for them to breathe. Ongoing fatigue and muscle weakness are other significant factors, as they are with other severe viral illnesses, which can limit a patient's capacity for work.

Long-term effects—economy

The economic damage of COVID-19 has come as the biggest shock the world has experienced in decades, despite extraordinary efforts by governments with stimulus packages to counteract the downturn. As a baseline forecast, global GDP in 2020 is expected to shrink by 5.2% using market exchange rate weights.[271] It will be the deepest global recession in decades, according to the author of the abovementioned feature story.

As of 30 July 2020, 42% of Australian businesses were accessing support measures such as wage subsidies, deferring loan repayments or renegotiating rental or lease arrangements, according to an Australian Bureau of Statistics media release.[272] One in 10 businesses reported that if support measures were no longer available, they would have to close their business.

Many people are being proactive in finding ways to continue trading, either online from home, or in the most severely affected hospitality industry, organising take-away meals as a substitute for in-room dining. COVID-19 is providing opportunities for creativity in developing new ways for service delivery which will, in many cases, continue.

As the end of June approached, more and more restrictions were eased. The government was keen for people to get back to work, 'It's time to come out of hibernation,' Prime Minister Scott Morrison said on *ABC News* in June 2020, 'and work on re-building the economy.' This, however, is proving to be easier said than done. The damage inflicted on some businesses is irreversible and unemployment in May 2020 reached a record high. Australia lost 227,000 jobs in May, increasing the unemployment rate to 7.1%. Unemployment in Australia has improved, especially during the last quarter of 2020. The Australian welfare payment JobKeeper has been instrumental in minimising the fallout from job losses but this support is due to end in March 2021 and things may change then.

While some Australian states are still reluctant to open their borders to all interstate travellers, others have done so, making life and work easier for many. But as soon as more community cases appear in a particular state, the borders slam shut again with homecoming travellers having to quarantine in hotels for two weeks at their own expense. The social distancing rules, being one-and-a-half metres from the next person and limiting group gatherings to one person per four square metres, together with stringent hygiene practices, are making it difficult for some businesses to operate, especially in the hospitality and tourism industries. International travel is still banned, but Qantas CEO Alan Joyce announced on 24 November 2020 that future overseas travellers will need to prove they have been vaccinated against COVID-19 before flying, if and when a safe and effective vaccine becomes widely available. Alan Joyce said that while Qantas is the first airline to enforce COVID-19 vaccination before overseas travel, he predicts it will be a common theme in the airline industry.[273]

Analysis of the full impact of COVID-19

It will be interesting, if and when an analysis is undertaken on the full impact of this coronavirus pandemic, to see just how many lives have been lost due to people diagnosed with COVID-19 and how many have been lost due to the mental health impacts it has caused based on fear. It will be no surprise to some if the numbers of the latter way surpass the former, at least on our home turf.

We all want this pandemic to end as soon as possible, either by the development of a safe and effective vaccine, safe treatments, including complementary and alternative therapies or by learning to live with it until it naturally dies out, medically and politically.

There has been a lot of fear generated around this pandemic but when people are armed with honest and reliable facts, they will be better equipped to do what needs to be done to defend and protect not only themselves and their loved ones but also their community and the whole of humanity.

It's not all doom and gloom on our little blue planet, even though, at times, it seems like it. There is hope for the future, but we just have to remain focused on our goals and use the power of intention to follow through, as suggested by Tony Robbins, motivational speaker, life coach and author of several books including *Awaken the Giant Within*. In this book, Tony describes how too many people shackle themselves with limiting beliefs, wanting to achieve goals but believing they are not capable of doing so. Tony understands the power of positive thinking and the potential people have for transformational change. He is a great believer in focusing on what we really want in life with a clear goal in mind, and purpose and meaning behind it. 'When you learn to focus your energy, amazing things happen,'[274] he said.

Key concepts

- There have been many positive aspects to emerge from the pandemic such as the improvement in homelessness, business innovation with the use of technology and education being digitalised and more affordable
- There will be a return to some manufacturing in Australia, making us less dependent on foreign imports
- The negative impacts have included increased domestic violence, child abuse, suicide and mental health issues
- Fear causes up to 90% of all disease
- There have been long-term effects on health and the economy

Pearl of wisdom

'Let me assert my firm belief that the only thing we have to fear, is fear itself—nameless, unreasoning, unjustified terror which paralyses needed efforts to convert retreat into advance.'

—Franklin D Roosevelt

CHAPTER 6

Pandemics in perspective

We had everything before us, we had nothing before us

Hope, Vision, Future

'Hold your head up high and don't be afraid of the dark,' I remind myself whilst preparing dinner on this humid December day. 'You'll Never Walk Alone' by Gerry and the Pacemakers is a soothing song and all people need comforting now. We've been through a lot in Australia during the last 12 months—drought, bushfires, floods and now, nine months later, coronavirus, COVID-19, is still causing havoc worldwide.

What's peculiar about this pandemic is that I have never known healthy people to be forced into quarantine. We have always isolated the sick, and this puzzles me. I am tired of stay-at-home mandates where people are unable to see family and friends in person and give them a hug. Virtual technology with FaceTime and Zoom is okay but isn't the same.

I enjoy problem-solving, researching if necessary, for answers. *Truth brings hope and knowledge is power*, I'm thinking while looking through my kitchen window. I decide not to be melancholy. Isolation loneliness and the threat of infection is one thing, but having bombs dropped nearby with nothing to eat would be much worse. I glance at a quote on my wall calendar, 'There are no hopeless situations, only people who have grown hopeless about them,' by Clare Luce.

With renewed determination, I walk to my bookshelf. I scan my volumes, looking for inspiration and the book *Tao Te Ching: The Ancient Book of Wisdom* by Lao Tzu, with commentary by Rory B Mackay,[275] catches my attention. I open the book and flick through the pages. What would Lao Tzu think about COVID-19 being genetically modified for gain-of-function from bat coronavirus in a bioweapons laboratory in Wuhan and allowed to escape, as indicated in the *Daily Telegraph* newspaper at the beginning of this pandemic? Was it deliberate or an accident and, if the latter, why was it covered up? Some people are caring and generous, but why does egotistical power and corruption have to reign supreme? Why is there so much injustice in the world? I wish humanity could work together in the spirit of kindness, goodwill, dignity and peace in a society that's connected to the natural world. Everyone should work harmoniously with nature, not against it. That's my dream.

I put the book aside and decide to research Taoism on the internet. The headline 'Taoism 101: Ancient Wisdom to Transform Your Life' immediately catches my attention. 'Become aware of the unity of all things and the interplay of opposites, the yin and yang,' I read. 'Instead of resisting problems and adversity, try letting things be. Be like water and find ways to flow around your obstacles with ease and grace.' I sit in my comfy chair and meditate for a while, thinking about water. If we agitate water in a pond it becomes muddy and we can't see a thing. If we simply allow it to settle, it will clear naturally and we will see everything.

Life won't be the same again and I wonder what the new 'normal' would be. I sigh. COVID-19 has changed the world; maybe the way we see the world needs to change too.

Although the world has changed immeasurably since the *Tao Te Ching* was written, its message is timeless and still as relevant today, as it was then. Society seems to have lost touch with the natural flow of life, prioritising the wantonness of wealth and material possessions with little interest in ethical and spiritual concerns.

A brief history of notable pandemics

Pandemics, pestilence and disease have been inflicted on human populations since the beginning of time, each with their own social and economic costs. To gain some perspective on the current situation, it may be useful to review the past.

Year	Disease	Number of deaths
1334	Black Death	30 to 50 million
1860s–1903	The modern plague	About 10 million
1889–1890	Russian Flu	About 1 million
1918–1919	Spanish Flu	50 to 100 million
1956–1958	Asian Flu	About 2 million
1968–1969	Hong Kong Flu	About 1 million
1976	Ebola	280
1981 (ongoing)	HIV/AIDS	About 32 million
2003	SARS	774
2009	Swine Flu	More than 200,000
2014	Ebola	More than 11,000
2019–20 (ongoing)	COVID-19	2,261,091 as at 02/02/2021

Source: https://theconversation.com/this-isnt-the-first-global-pandemic-and-it-wont-be-the-last-heres-what-weve-learnt-from-4-others-throughout-history-136231. [Updated]: COVID-19 Coronavirus Pandemic, Worldometer, https://www.worldometers.info/coronavirus/

Other information

Bubonic plague.

Originated in China and spread to Europe along trade routes.

Bubonic plague.

Started in China and then spread to Hong Kong by 1894.

Influenza A.

The pandemic was first recorded in Russia and then spread through Europe, Asia and reached the USA.

Influenza A (H1N1).

Estimated to have infected over 500 million people worldwide.

Influenza A (H2N2)

Originated in China and spread to Singapore, Hong Kong and the USA.

Influenza A (H3N2).

Started in Hong Kong and then spread through Asia, Australia, Europe and the USA.

The first recorded outbreak of the Ebola virus [occurred near the Ebola River in Zaire, now the Democratic Republic of Congo (DRC) from where it spread to other African countries].[276]

Human immunodeficiency virus (HIV), Develops into acquired immunodeficiency syndrome (AIDS).

Thought to have originated in West Africa in the early 20th century, discovered in the US in 1981, has spread globally.

Viral respiratory illness (coronavirus).

The initial outbreak was reported in southern China and then quickly moved to Hong Kong and other countries.

Influenza A (H1N1).

WHO estimates around 18,500 deaths, but other research suggests a death toll of over 200,000 people.

Over 28,000 cases of Ebola reported.

The worst-hit countries were Liberia, Sierra Leone and Guinea in West Africa.

Viral respiratory illness (coronavirus).

The initial outbreak in China's Hubei province, before quickly spreading throughout Asia, then to Iran, parts of Europe and eventually worldwide.

The two pandemics that stand out during the last century, with millions of deaths, are the Spanish Flu of 1918–19 with 50 to 100 million deaths and HIV/AIDS in 1981 (ongoing) which has been attributed to causing about 32 million deaths. Just how many deaths COVID-19 will cause before it dies out is the big unknown, but one needs to be mindful that the rules of infectiology and reporting have become increasingly rubbery over time distorting the figures. As of 2 February 2021, there have been 104,342,713 identified cases of COVID-19 with 2,261,091 deaths and 76,108,618 recoveries, according to *Worldometer* coronavirus pandemic information.[277]

The Spanish Flu

It's not clear exactly where the Spanish Flu began, but it appears that it wasn't in Spain. Researchers have suggested France, China, Britain and the United States as the potential birthplace. Wherever this flu outbreak originated, it was officially reported in Madrid in the spring of 1918, which led to this pandemic being called the Spanish Flu.

Researchers have yet to discover why that particular H1N1 strain was so lethal, particularly in the 16 weeks from mid-September to mid-December 1918.[278] The similarity between the Spanish Flu and COVID-19 is that they both wreak havoc on the immune system by triggering a cytokine storm—an overreaction of the body's immune system. The difference between these two diseases is the former was more prevalent among young adults, and the latter, older adults.

During the Spanish Flu, the poor people were considered to be vectors, spreading infection to the better-off classes and, during the COVID-19 pandemic, that situation is reversed, where the globally mobile affluent people have spread the disease to the 'favelas and the poor'.[279]

The Spanish Flu Experiment

During the Spanish Flu in 1919, scientists at the US Public Health Service and others were interested in trying to determine how this disease spread so widely and rapidly around the world and conducted experiments on healthy volunteers from the US Navy.

In the landmark study published in the *Journal of the American Medical Association*, 2 August 1919,[280] scientists collected mixtures from the throat and noses of selected influenza cases and administered these to 10 young healthy US Navy volunteers. They drew blood from influenza patients and transferred it to the volunteers. They collected mucus swabs from influenza patients and, after filtering them to exclude larger molecules such as bacteria, injected the filtrate into the volunteers. The volunteers mingled with the influenza patients, were coughed on and breathed upon and shook hands. Not one volunteer became sick from all these interventions. This experiment was repeated with another 50 volunteers with the same result.

As Dr Rosenau commented in the above referred-to article, 'We entered the [Spanish Flu] outbreak with a notion that we knew the cause of the disease, and were quite sure we knew how it was transmitted from person to person. Perhaps, if we have learnt anything, it is that we are not quite sure what we know about the disease.' This is a reminder of the Socratic paradox derived from Plato's account of the Greek philosopher Socrates, 'The only thing that I know is that I know nothing.'

HIV/AIDS

It's believed that the human immunodeficiency virus (HIV) originated in Kinshasa in the Democratic Republic of Congo around 1920 when this disease crossed species from chimpanzees to humans, moving to Haiti in the 1960s and San Francisco in the 1970s and spreading to other continents worldwide during the 1980s.

HIV damages the immune system, leading to acquired immunodeficiency syndrome (AIDS) when the body loses its ability to fight infection and disease. It's estimated that over 30 million people have died of HIV/AIDS. This virus can now be successfully treated with drugs that slow its progression, especially if treatment is commenced in the early stages of infection, but a cure is yet to be found.

How do pandemics end?

There are two types of 'endings' for pandemics—the medical ending when the death rates plummet and herd immunity is established, and the social ending, when the intensity of fear about the disease diminishes.[281] 'When people ask when will this end, they are asking about the social ending,' said Dr Jeremy Greene, a historian of medicine at Johns Hopkins University.

So, in effect, a disease can end when people pay less attention to it and go about their normal business as much as possible; when they get tired of panic mode and learn to live with the disease or it dies out naturally, medically and politically. Mr Allan Brandt, a Harvard historian said in 'How Pandemics End' in *The New York Times*, 'As we have seen in the debate about opening the economy, many questions about the so-called end are determined not by medical and public health data, but by socio-political processes.'[282]

Australian Prime Minister Scott Morrison made his view clear. He said any attempt to eliminate COVID-19 entirely in Australia 'would come at too high a cost, both to the economy and the welfare of those living under lockdown'.[283]

What we have learnt from previous pandemics

As noted in 'Silver Lining: Could COVID-19 lead to a better future', pandemics are often an instigating factor for social and political reform.

The Plague or Black Death of the 14ᵗʰ century

The bubonic plague, known as the Black Death, in the 14ᵗʰ century, was responsible for the death of one-third of the world population. It's believed to have started in China and moved west in caravans along trade routes. It resulted in 'improved working and living conditions for low-income workers of that era, which in turn led to healthier diets and better resistance to later reoccurrences of the disease'.[284]

Widespread death caused labour shortages, leading to higher wages, cheaper land, better living conditions and increased freedoms for the lower class. By improving their diet and living conditions, people in this feudal society were able to build a stronger immune system that protected them from further outbreaks of the bubonic plague.

This pandemic, reported to have killed between 30 and 50 million people at a time when the world population was relatively small, catalysed enormous societal, economic, artistic and cultural reforms in medieval Europe, becoming a turning point in history, with enduring impacts. During this time, people began to question rigid beliefs around structure, traditions and orthodox religions. England and France were so overwhelmed by this disease that they had to call off their war at the time, proving that disease can end physical wars.

The Spanish Flu of 1918

This pandemic of recent history had devastating consequences, killing millions of people worldwide, and was difficult to combat. Strategies such as the wearing of facemasks and bans on mass gatherings were utilised to prevent the spread of this disease, building on previous success with controlling tuberculosis, cholera and other infectious diseases. The public health system throughout the developed world during this time was in its infancy and only the middle class and wealthy people could afford to visit a doctor.

This pandemic spurred the development of public health systems in the western world as scientists and governments realised just how quickly viral pandemics of this magnitude could spread. A good public health system is the best defence against disease.[285]

Lessons from the sun

Another lesson that should have been learnt from the 1918–1919 Spanish flu and, to date, hasn't, is the benefit of open-air treatment—fresh air and sunshine. Overcrowding and poor ventilation are the two main factors that contributed to poor outcomes for most patients, in both situations, the Spanish Flu and COVID-19, with patients dying not from viral infection but from pneumonia and other complications induced by the cytokine storm.

In the US city of Boston in 1918, medical staff decided to adopt a different form of treatment. The state guard set up an emergency tent hospital and took the worst cases among sailors on ships in Boston Harbour and gave them as much fresh air as possible by putting them in tents. When weather permitted, they were taken out of their tents and placed in the sun. 'Apparently, the fatality of hospital cases was reduced from 40 per cent to about 13 per cent by the treatment.'[286]   Also, the benefits of fresh air and sunshine were not limited to the patients. The same journal article further states, 'An invaluable incident to this treatment is the fact that in the open air, the immunity of the nurses and physicians is enormously increased, leaving them to carry out the great amount of work confronting them.'

Dr Richard Hobday, PhD, an internationally recognised researcher and author commented in 'Coronavirus and the Sun: A Lesson from the 1918 Influenza Pandemic':

'Put simply, medics found that severely ill flu patients nursed outdoors recovered better than those treated indoors. A combination of fresh air and sunlight seems to have prevented deaths among patients; and infections among medical staff [cited in 'The Open-Air Treatment of PANDEMIC INFLUENZA']. There is scientific support for this. Research shows that outdoor air is a natural disinfectant. Fresh air can kill the flu virus and other harmful germs. Equally, sunlight is germicidal and there is now evidence it can kill the flu virus.'[287]

Many scientific researchers over time have highlighted the beneficial effects of fresh air and sunshine when treating disease. 'Among the first advocates of what was later to become known as the "open-air method" was the English physician John Coakley Lettsom (1744-1815), who exposed children suffering from tuberculosis to sea air and sunshine at the Royal Sea Bathing Hospital in Kent, England, in 1791.'[288]

HIV/AIDS of the 20ᵗʰ century

This pandemic, which was at its peak between 1983 and 1991, taught us the value of a well-designed public health campaign and the importance of de-stigmatising disease, allowing people to feel that they could be tested safely and be supported during the disease process.

The initial failure of politics to support this cohort of the population led to millions of deaths before a breakthrough treatment was discovered that prevented HIV from developing into AIDS. People were not cured of the virus, but the advent of a political movement that funded science, treatment, prevention, civil rights protection and health care access was instrumental in reforming a public health system that had failed millions of people.

The author of an opinion piece published in *The Hill* suggests there is much we can learn to forge our way ahead in the COVID-19 crisis, in particular, 'three things that must prevail: sound policy formed by experts in close alignment with science and facts; mature politics by leaders who set aside ideology, take responsibility and unite us under comprehensive legislation; and public knowledge of facts, not spins on stories that propagate more confusion and distrust'.[289]

Severe Acute Respiratory Syndrome (SARS) of 2002–2003

SARS should have taught us that timely and truthful information sharing is paramount in preventing the spread of infectious diseases. We have the technology for this to happen and it should be possible.

'SARS was a catalyst for change in China where the government invested in enhanced surveillance systems that facilitate the real time collection and communication of infectious diseases and syndromes from emergency departments back to a centralised government database,' according to Justin Denholm from *SBS News*.[290] This author further states that the information technology and knowledge gained from SARS allowed the prompt isolation and genetic sequencing of the SARS-CoV-2 so it could be shared globally in a timely manner.

Lessons we can learn from the COVID-19 pandemic

Sometimes the greatest lessons in life are found from the greatest problems, and COVID-19 is no exception. The unpleasant experiences that we have endured during this pandemic should awaken our thinking to seek a new way forward. Some of these adjustments may include focusing on simple living, the importance of hygiene and learning how to be content alone, slowing down and learning to appreciate nature. Other major lessons we should learn from this pandemic are as follows:

The interdependence of human and planetary life

Human health and the health of our communities and environment need to be considered as a holistic entity. Mother Nature has had a lot to say in recent years, and we haven't been listening. As a result, she has been ramping up the intensity of natural disasters such as droughts, bushfires and floods in various parts of the world to get our attention.

We, as human beings, are just one part of the ecosystem and, for that system to be healthy, all plants, animals and people living both in a particular area and more broadly, need to live and work well together, accommodating the complex relationships that exist between them, their communities and the environment in which they live.

Truth in reporting

Transparency is key to building trust and this requires honest and open communications in science, government, bureaucracy, the media and people from all walks of life. People generally are becoming more aware and know when the wool is being pulled over their eyes, causing them to sometimes become suspicious and distrusting of what they are being told. If we are supposed to be all in this together, then let us be open and honest with each other and share the truth, no matter what it might be, rather than have the 'thought police' make judgements as to what people should be told.

Cooperation and collaboration

Global threats require a global response and cooperation between nations, and similarly between states in different countries. Instead of national and international cooperation during this pandemic, we have often seen strategic rivalry and fragmenting power games played out with serious consequences across all levels of society.

'United we stand, divided we fall' is well worth remembering, not only in times of crisis but in all areas and avenues of life. There needs to be greater emphasis on global responsibility and stewardship to build stronger, more collaborative bonds within and between all nations across the globe.

The importance of the private sector

Medicare, the Australian universal healthcare system, was introduced in 1984 by the Australian Labor Party and has been of great benefit to all citizens, but this and other public services can't be sustained by a welfare state where a large percentage of the working population is receiving government payments such as JobKeeper, as is becoming evident in Australia.

Extraordinary times may call for extraordinary measures, but we can't keep depending on the public purse for everything. Australian values are enshrined in the National Anthem with one of them being 'wealth for toil' not 'wealth from welfare'. Sadly, many people prefer not to work, but instead receive welfare. People need jobs, but they also need to be prepared to work when jobs are available.

In Australia, farmers are having to sacrifice their crops and plough produce back into the ground because of the scarcity of people willing to work. This will ultimately lead to a shortage of food supply and an increase in prices, causing additional financial stress for all people across the board. There should be more emphasis on Work for the Dole, an Australian government initiative that is a form of 'workfare' or work-based welfare. It was trialled in 1997 and permanently enacted in 1998 as a mutual obligation requirement for receiving government payments such as JobSeeker.[291]

Many private companies have retooled their manufacturing capacity to produce urgently needed medical equipment and supplies for the benefit of all. Governments can't do everything, especially without tax revenue from the private sector.

Elderly people should not suffer in nursing homes

If there is a lesson that should be learnt from this pandemic, it is rectifying the generally deplorable state of nursing homes and the tragedy of so many residents dying of COVID-19 in these facilities. Unlike the majority of people in society, these people are often helpless, vulnerable and have few resources to protect themselves in times of crisis. There is a systemic failure of governments and aged care sectors worldwide to adequately cater for people in this demographic.

Our parents and grandparents residing in nursing homes or residential care facilities are esteemed citizens who have raised families, paid their taxes and fought for their country. They deserve a much better standard of living in their golden years than the meagre rations and lack of dignity and respect with which they are being afforded. These failings have been bubbling away for years and are typically brushed aside and ignored. We can only hope that this situation has raised enough conscious thought to bring about radical change.

'Most Important Coronavirus Statistic: 42% of US deaths are from 0.6% of the population'[292] is a sobering disclosure of elder deaths and it's tragic to think that this can be largely prevented by the methods outlined in this book, such as improving diet and nutrition, and in particular, maintaining a high vitamin D blood serum level. This group of people is particularly at risk of vitamin D deficiency because they generally spend little time outside in the sunshine, and even if they have sufficient sun exposure, they have a diminished ability to convert it to vitamin D.[293]

Staying connected while disconnected

Even though social distancing, attention to hygiene and regular handwashing may be with us for some time as a public health measure to prevent the spread of disease and 'we're all in this together', it's important to understand that while we can feel somewhat disconnected in our 'new normal' society, we need to stay connected as best we can. This applies not only to the pandemic but what we can do to improve our connectedness in the future.

Advances in technology, while not always our friend, especially with personal scams and cyber attacks, can be helpful with keeping in touch with our family and friends via, for example, FaceTime, Skype and Zoom. Loneliness has become a major concern, particularly amongst elderly people who may not be as savvy with new technology, either through lack of understanding or distrust of this medium of social exchange. There's nothing wrong with the telephone, and a quick hello and chat can make a world of difference to someone feeling isolated and lonely in a shrinking, secular world.

We should be promoting a wellness model of healthcare

COVID-19 is a wake-up call highlighting major flaws in our society and calling (or forcing) us to take action and remedy these situations.

Our current medical model of healthcare is based on treating disease with drugs, surgery, radiation and other prescribed therapies, and this is a profitable industry guided by science. But unfortunately, as we have seen, sometimes the science becomes corrupt and cannot be trusted.

If the medical model was changed to focus more on prevention—living a healthier lifestyle through diet, nutrition, exercise, rest and relaxation, lifestyle diseases would become virtually extinct. Millions of people would be either immune from COVID-19 and other diseases, or if they did become infected, they would not be so vulnerable to the consequences. The medical model of healthcare, also known as the sickness model, wouldn't collapse but would be balanced with a wellness model integrating both sides of the healthcare system, sickness and wellness for more holistic outcomes.

Artificial Intelligence and Big Data

Another example of what we can learn from this pandemic is in the area of Artificial Intelligence (AI) and how Big Data and AI will play a key role in manifesting our forward trajectory, whether that means sliding further down the rabbit hole to a dystopian future or unlocking a type of utopian heaven on earth … and the choice is ours.

What a dystopian future will look like under AI surveillance

The Chinese social credit system

The future of western civilisation is hanging precariously in the balance with the COVID-19 pandemic. For the first time in history, Big Data and AI have joined together with China's social credit system to enable governments to monitor everyone all the time. This social credit system was unveiled by the Chinese Communist Party (CCP) in 2014 to build a database that monitors individual, corporate and government behaviour across a country in real-time. According to the author of an article in *The South China Morning Post*, the trustworthiness of individuals, companies and government entities is assessed and given a social credit score, rewarding those who have a high rating and punishing those with low scores.[294]

Big Data is being used to build a society where individuals and organisations follow prescribed laws or pay the penalty if they don't. This social credit system is designed to control and coerce people in a gigantic social engineering experiment and is described as 'a "digital dictatorship" and a "dystopian nightmare straight out of [TV show] Black Mirror",[295] a British dystopian science fiction anthology.

According to an article published in *Global Research* and reported on social media, the reason for the two-month night-time curfew in Melbourne during hard lockdown from early August 2020 was to allow elements of the Chinese social credit system to be installed in secrecy under cover of darkness. It was claimed that planes from the Chinese province of Guangdong were landing in the night carrying equipment related to 5G and the Chinese social credit system.[296] Understandably, curfews may have been necessary in some areas of the US to control civil unrest, but no such violent protests were taking place in Melbourne. But perhaps the virus is more virulent after dark!

The Internet of Things (IoT) is a key aspect of AI and surveillance. It interconnects between various 'things' and other entities such as people or applications using smart technology. 'There are multiple risks associated with certain technological applications, since all technologies used by governments in the control and fight of the pandemic can be used for surveillance and pose undeniable threats to privacy, individual freedoms, and democracy.'[297]

Lawmakers have passed legislation while we have been hiding in lockdown 'ordering phone carriers to continuously track geolocations of all smartphone users'.[298] Big Data is being used inappropriately by surveillance capitalists where our privacy details are being mined for the benefit of third parties and our civil liberties have been trampled upon in the name of public health.

The Quick Response (QR) Code

The Quick Response (QR) code, a scannable square matrix barcode first designed in 1994 for the automotive industry in Japan, facilitates electronic check-ins at cafés and restaurants, etc, and the data is outsourced to registration platforms that are often owned by companies specialising in collecting data, with some of them operating under opaque rules about how the information is stored and used. 'There are concerns that the data could potentially be resold, used for identity fraud or to track a person's location and social groups, and employed in micro-targeted advertising for misinformation campaigns.'[299]

A malicious URL may be embedded in the code that takes the user to a site where malware can be installed on their mobile device and share sensitive information with cybercriminals. This allows hackers and cybercriminals to make calendar, contacts and credit card information available to criminal networks, steal Facebook, Google and other passwords and post information without the owner's knowledge or permission, track the owner's location for criminal purposes and infect the mobile device with malicious software that can disable it.[300] Mobile devices are unlikely to carry any security software, making them a prime target for hackers and cybercriminals.

Altering the course of political elections

Data misappropriation has also been used to sway political elections such as 'Cambridge Analytica's mission to transform surveys and Facebook data into a political messaging weapon.'[301] Highly sophisticated micro-targeting operations are used, taking advantage of people's emotions. Their behaviour and psychological profiles are obtained from their internet footprint and Facebook and similar platforms are gold mines for this information. Different voters receive different messages based on predictions about their susceptibility to different arguments. 'The paranoid received ads with messages based around fear. People with a conservative predisposition received ads with arguments based on tradition and community.'[302]

Data is gold. The more information big data companies can mine from social media, tracking and surveillance platforms such as what people like, how they think and where they frequent, the more AI they have at their disposal. 'Whoever becomes the leader in this [AI] sphere will become the ruler of the world,' said Russian President Vladimir Putin,[303] and his views are shared by national security leaders in the US, China and other countries. Elon Musk commented in the abovementioned article, that in his opinion, the grapple for AI superiority will be the most likely cause of World War III.

Injectable hydrogel biosensor to detect infections

Profusa, a Silicon Valley company with ties to the US military-industrial complex, pioneered an injectable hydrogel biosensor that will integrate with human tissue to continuously monitor body chemistry and detect early signs of infection in the event of an outbreak of disease. In news provided by *Profusa Inc*, the company states, 'The RTI DARPA SIGMA+ funded effort is based on evaluating monitoring platforms including Profusa's first-of-its-kind, minimally invasive injectable biosensor technology, the Lumee™ Oxygen Platform, to measure tissue oxygen levels as a potential indicator of human response to infection or exposure.'[304] This technology can also continuously transmit actionable, medical-grade data for personal, medical and other use.

Hydrogel chip will connect you to the internet

The injectable hydrogel biosensor will emit various signals with the following properties and capabilities:

'The sensor has two parts. One is a 3mm string of hydrogel, a material whose network of polymer chains is used in some contact lenses and other implants. Inserted under the skin with a syringe, the string includes a specifically engineered molecule that sends a fluorescent signal outside the body when the body begins to fight an infection. The other part is an electronic component attached to the skin [similar to a Fitbit or other smartwatch]. It sends light through the skin, detects the fluorescent signal and generates another signal that the wearer can send to a doctor, website, etc. It's like a blood lab on the skin that can pick up the body's response to illness before the presence of other symptoms, like coughing.'[305]

This early identification system aims to detect new disease outbreaks in the community, including biological attacks and pandemics up to three weeks in advance of the current public health network data system. Profusa hopes to gain FDA approval for their injectable biosensor in early 2021, opening the door for widespread surveillance of human body systems. Access to every person's bloodstream is necessary for this scheme to succeed on a worldwide scale, which is possible if mandatory vaccination is enforced, as discussed in the above referred-to article.

COVID-19 mRNA vaccines contain hydrogel

The Profusa biosensor and the COVID-19 mRNA vaccines are similar in that they both utilise hydrogel in their delivery system.[306] The hydrogel invented by the US Defense Advanced Research Projects Agency (DARPA) involves nanotechnology. 'This "bioelectronic interface" is part of the COVID-19 mRNA vaccines' delivery system,' as stated in the abovementioned article. Using hydrogel in the COVID-19 mRNA vaccines such as those developed by Pfizer and Moderna may be one way to get a large percentage of the global population trapped in the 'net' ready for AI manipulation.

mRNA vaccines are not a vaccine but a medical device

Dr David Martin, a medical and legal expert with an impressive bio that can be viewed at his website,[307] challenges what we are supposed to believe about the mRNA vaccines—that they are approximately 95% effective against COVID-19. David is adamant that the mRNA vaccines are not a vaccine in the legal definition of the term, but a medical device designed to stimulate the cell into becoming a pathogen creator.[308] An excerpt from this video is as follows:

'We need to be really clear. We're using the term "vaccine" to sneak this thing under the public health exemptions. This is not a vaccine. This is a mRNA packaged in a fat envelope, that is delivered to a cell. It is a medical device designed to stimulate the human cell into becoming a pathogen creator. It is not a vaccine. Vaccines actually are a legally defined term, and they're a legally defined term under public health law; they're a legally defined term under the CDC and FDA standards. And a vaccine specifically has to stimulate both an immunity within the person who is receiving it, but it also has to disrupt transmission. And that is not what this is. They have been abundantly clear in saying that the mRNA strand that is going into the cell is not to stop transmission. It is a treatment. But if it was discussed as a treatment, it would not get the sympathetic ear of the public health authorities, because the people would say, well, what other treatments are there?'

The gene-based DNA and mRNA vaccines are a great potential danger as they can alter a person's DNA, in the event of the former, or cause autoimmune reactions in both instances, the prospects of which are simply terrifying, according to Dr Karina Reiss and Dr Sucharit Bhakdi, authors of *Corona False Alarm: Facts and Figures*. 'No gene-based vaccine has ever received approval for human use, and the present coronavirus vaccines have not undergone preclinical testing as normally required by international regulations.'

Thousands of volunteers have subjected themselves to clinical trials of gene-based and other vaccines and have not been informed of all the potential risks. It simply beggars belief how some countries prohibit the use of genetically modified foods and oppose cruelty to animals, yet genetic experiments are being conducted on humans with these vaccines and safety regulations have been bypassed to expedite rollout. This has been allowed to happen because of the suspension of human rights laws under emergency powers due to the COVID-19 pandemic. All this is taking place because of a virus that, medically, has an infection fatality rate no worse than the flu but politically, it's another story—power, corruption and greed reign supreme.

In another interesting rabbit hole twist, Profusa has received funding from the US National Institutes of Health (NIH), a government agency, to develop their tissue integrated biosensors. The Moderna vaccine is being developed in partnership with the NIH. Dr Anthony Fauci is director of the NIAID, which comes under the umbrella of the NIH, and he owns a patent or patents in the mRNA Moderna/NIH vaccine. As discussed in chapter three, this conflict of interest has been allowed under the provisions of the US *Bayh-Dole Act* that gave government workers the right to patent their discoveries. All this began with GOF research funded by the NIH under the directorship of Dr Fauci and moved to a BSL-4 laboratory in Wuhan, China, when the Obama administration ceased funding due to its potential risks, as discussed in chapter two.

When science fiction becomes reality

While Profusa claims that their injectable biosensor technology will empower individuals to monitor their body chemistry in ways that will transform the management of personal health and disease, there is also the capability that such nanotechnology 'could theoretically be used to make mind-control systems, invisible and mobile eavesdropping services, or unimaginably horrific tools of torture.'[309] The author of the previously mentioned article, 'Injectable Biochip for SARS-CoV-2 Detection Near FDA Approval' states, 'If your cellphone can receive information from your body, what information can your body receive from it, or other sources, and what effects might such transmissions have on your physical functioning and psychological health? So far, such crucial questions have not been answered, and they must be considering the nightmarish possibilities' such as the potential for people to be punished under the CCP social credit system, or something similar.

Elon Musk is terrified of AI taking over the world

As far-fetched as the prospects of AI may seem to the average person, this technology is available now and many aspects of it will be implemented whether we agree to it or not. Even Elon Musk, business entrepreneur, industrial designer and engineer, is extremely concerned about where AI is heading and what could potentially mean the end of our species with this technology. In his view, 'human beings could become the equivalent of "house cats" to new AI overlords [and has] repeatedly called for regulation and caution when it comes to new AI technology.'[310] In a *New York Times* interview cited in this article, Elon said, 'Just the nature of the AI that they're building is one that crushes all humans at all games. I mean, it's basically the plotline in *WarGames*.' Elon has also commented that AI has the potential to become superior to human intelligence within the next five years, even if it's not immediately apparent. 'That doesn't mean that everything goes to hell in five years,' he said. 'It just means that things get unstable or weird.' Elon Musk believes that people generally underestimate the capability of AI and even the smartest of people refuse to believe that any computer could be smarter than them.

What about privacy?

As far as privacy is concerned with AI, many questions remain unanswered. With all the additional mass surveillance and biological data supposedly required to protect us against SARS-CoV-2 and any future pandemics, a massively increased bandwidth in cellphone and Wi-Fi networks is required and this could be the reason why governments around the world are rushing to instal 5G networks and why the CCP was very keen to instal their Huawei 5G network in Australia.

The Great Reset

Another arm of AI is the Great Reset, discussed in chapter two. This is the technocratic fascist vision of Professor Klaus Schwab, founder and executive chairman of the World Economic Forum, to monitor and control the world through digital surveillance. At the World Economic Forum's Great Reset Initiative held in June 2020, discussions centred around stripping all people of their privately owned assets. In Klaus Schwab's book, *COVID-19: The Great Reset*, industry leaders and decision-makers are urged to make good use of the pandemic and not let the crisis go to waste. Dr Mercola has the following comment:

'At this point, it should be obvious for anyone paying attention that the pandemic is being prolonged and exaggerated for a reason, and it's not because there's concern for life. Quite the contrary … It should also be clear that most if not all pandemic restrictions to freedom are meant to become permanent. In other words, these past nine months have been a preview of the world the technocratic elite wants to implement as part of the new social economic order.'[311]

We need to act now, not later

In an article published in *The Conversation*, the author refers to AI machines such as robots having human-level intelligence with advanced computational powers far superior to their human creators and envisions such a reality somewhere between 2029 and the end of the century. 'When they do [arrive], there is a great and natural concern that we won't be able to control them,'[312] he said. 'The next decade or so represents a critical period. There is an opportunity to create safe and efficient AGI [artificial general intelligence] systems that can have far reaching benefits to society and humanity. At the same time, a business-as-usual approach in which we play catch-up with rapid technological advances could contribute to the extinction of the human race. The ball is in our court, but it won't be for much longer.'

A utopian future

An alternative to this privacy deprivation and data mining measure concerning the QR code is to utilise the system that the United Kingdom and New Zealand have adopted and that is having a QR code program that allows visitors to 'anonymously register' that they have been to a location such as a café, restaurant, football game or CWA meeting without having their data stored and used by third parties for potentially criminal purposes. In this situation, the information is stored locally on the person's device only, like a personal diary, and not outsourced to third parties. Privacy is better protected. If a person tests positive to

COVID-19, health authorities can access encrypted data stored on individual phones and issue a public health alert about the patient's movements.

We can choose to either passively succumb to the tyranny of China's social credit system and other game-changers such as sentient robots bossing us around and allow Big Data and AI to determine our future, or alternatively, people can actively seek a golden age of empowerment and equality using people power to enforce change. In the latter scenario, ordinary citizens could take back their power and reclaim their privacy and civil liberties by insisting that all biometric data seized for surveillance and tracking to monitor compliance with lockdown guidelines be returned to the people for their own purposes in the form of protected Trusted Execution Environment (TEE) technologies, enabling only the user to access their personal biometric information. A TEE environment is a secure area of a main computer processor where the code and data are protected for confidentiality and integrity, meaning that the information collected cannot be seen or changed by another party outside the TEE environment.[313] Collecting information in a TEE environment will empower individual owners of personal data to better monitor their health and alert them to possible risks in their near vicinity, promoting compassion, empowerment and personal responsibility instead of finger-pointing, disempowerment and judgement.

The COVID-19 pandemic could be a catalyst for a universal movement to disallow mass surveillance in any form.

Learning to be adaptable

Pandemics can teach us valuable lessons on adaptability—how we can live our lives more in tune with ourselves and each other and with our natural environment. In 'What Hard Times Teach Us: 5 pandemic inspired lessons that will make you better for the long term', the author offers the following suggestions:

Finding perspective—have patience and appreciate the longer view.

Resilience and response—learn to be adaptable and creative.

Community—stay connected and be grateful for everyday things.

Managing yourself—exercise self-discipline and self-care.

Finding happiness—be optimistic; hard times can be the catalyst for new habits, behaviours and lessons.[314]

How COVID-19 may reshape the balance of power

The international balance of power is a fluid entity shifting like sands through the hourglass of time as countries rise and fall in their political, economic and military strength on the global stage.

World War II resulted in the defeat of Germany and Italy by Britain, France and the United States of America, which led to the rise of the US as the major authority in the international arena and the decline of Britain as the top-ranking leader in terms of military and economic power.

The USSR attempted to seize supremacy for themselves during the Cold War between 1946 and 1991 when the United States, the Soviet Union and their respective allies were locked in a long, tense conflict characterised by an aggressive arms race, proxy wars and ideological bids for world dominance. India and other Asian/African nations refused to be drawn into this skirmish and chose the middle ground of non-alliance. India was regarded as a balance of power between the US and the USSR and peace-keeping negotiations between these countries resulted in substantial economic aid from the US and defence assistance from the USSR.

The US maintained its superiority as the world's foremost leader during the Cold War, but the sands started to shift in 1972 with the formal entry of Communist China into the international system after US President Nixon's historic visit to China in early 1972. This visit, aimed at ending 20 years of frosty relations between the two countries, was considered an important strategic and diplomatic occasion, marking the resumption of harmonious relations between the US and mainland China after years of political isolation. The entry of China into the international alliance was viewed as a countermeasure to contain the political aspirations of the USSR as a potential world leader.

Since President Nixon's inaugural visit, Communist China has started to slowly emerge as a force in world politics, in alignment with the exponential growth in its economy. This has been most notable in recent years under the dictatorship of President Xi Jinping when the influence of the Chinese Communist Party started posing a challenge, not only for the US in its role as global leader but also the Western world with the incremental erosion of democratic values that we have allowed.

The outbreak of COVID-19 in China during December 2019 and its rapid spread to the US, Europe and the rest of the world, has caused some heated discussions about possible changes in the international balance of power. A disease of this magnitude, with its 'no passport requirements', has shown how quickly a country can be brought to its knees, despite its political, economic and military might. COVID-19 has proved that physical warfare is unnecessary—biological warfare can achieve a desired agenda and wreak just as much havoc, if not more, than military battles.

Although China has suffered considerably with this disease, it seems to have emerged less scathed than other countries, if we believe what we have been told. The CCP has been manoeuvring itself, largely under the radar, for political supremacy, and their exponential rise in economic status and advances in technology have allowed them to achieve this.

US/China relations have eroded in recent years with similar misgivings realised by other world leaders. Subterfuge, imposed bans on selective imports into China and cyber attacks from this regime have been rendered against the Western world.

The CCP may want to shift the international balance of power from the US to China and appoint themselves as the preeminent leader on the global stage, but these ideals have been seriously jeopardised due to lack of trust and transparency. 'More than the pandemic, global dissatisfaction and anger about the suppression of COVID-19 by the Chinese leadership has resulted in a serious trust deficit and consequently its legitimacy in the world. A survey carried out by Pew Research Centre points to China's unpopularity hitting historic highs in 14 advanced economies in the world, thereby affecting its standing in the world.'[315]

Many people predict that the US will maintain its power base and continue to lead the western world, despite the setback it experienced in recent times with the negative consequences of COVID-19 and the destabilising nature of the political tug-of-war between the US and China.

Joe Biden was sworn in as the 46th President of the United States of America on 20 January 2021 in Washington DC with Kamala Harris the first female Vice-President. It will be interesting to see how Joe Biden steers his country in relation to the political aspirations of China and how much that will affect the Western world. Maybe he will negotiate a truce between the US and China and the US will maintain its supremacy in the world with the balance of power in their favour. Or maybe Joe Biden will lean more to the left and embrace the communist ideals of the CCP as his way of restoring peace.

Or maybe, as former Australian Prime Minister, Kevin Rudd, has suggested, 'The uncomfortable truth is that China and the United States are both likely to emerge from this crisis significantly diminished … and the result will be a continued slow but steady drift toward international anarchy across everything from international security to trade to pandemic management.'[316]

The story of the Chinese farmer

As this book comes to a close, the story of Taoist tradition about a farmer who had worked his crops for many years comes to mind.

A farmer and his family in ancient China owned a horse. His neighbours said how lucky he was to have such a fine horse to pull his plough through the fields. The farmer said, 'Maybe yes, maybe no.'

One day the horse broke through the gate and ran away. His neighbours came around to lament his terrible loss, saying it was a terrible bit of bad luck. The farmer said, 'Maybe yes, maybe no.'

Days later, the horse returned to the farm along with seven wild horses. His neighbours came around to exclaim his remarkable good fortune, saying, 'Now you are rich!' The farmer said, 'Maybe yes, maybe no.'

A few weeks later, the farmer's son was training the new wild horses, fell off one and broke his leg. The neighbours came around to commiserate his misfortune and said, 'What bad luck! The farmer replied, 'Maybe yes, maybe no.'

The next week the army came around, taking all the able-bodied young men from the village to fight in the war. The farmer's son with the broken leg was left behind. The neighbours now lamented the loss of their sons and commented on how lucky the farmer was to have his son.

The moral of this story

You never know what the consequence of misfortune or good fortune will be. In this story, at first glance, it appears that the farmer was ambivalent and didn't care about anything. But there's a deeper meaning. It suggests that no single event, in and of itself, can be judged good or bad, right or wrong, lucky or unlucky because, when one door closes, another one opens that may offer even greater opportunities than those experienced before.

Benjamin Franklin, US statesman, diplomat, writer and inventor said, 'Out of adversity comes opportunity.' Many people have lost their jobs due to COVID-19 and it's understandable that they're suffering terrible hardship. But in the future, new positions may present themselves that lead to better personal and financial rewards, so it pays to cultivate detachment and fortitude as a way of experiencing more equanimity in the face of ever-changing circumstances.

Life is never static, things change, we change and we have to adapt. We must adapt to nature because nature can't change for us. If we try to fight the natural forces, they will overcome us. The Chinese farmer understood this. He didn't concern himself with future events, what may or may not happen, because he accepted that change was inevitable, for better or for worse, and that many events were beyond his control. He not only accepted that; he was at peace with it.

Key concepts
- There have been many pandemics and epidemics throughout human history with two stand-out ones being the Spanish Flu and HIV/AIDS
- There are two ways that pandemics end—the medical ending where herd immunity is established and the social ending when fear about the disease diminishes
- What we have learnt from previous pandemics and what we can learn from COVID-19
- Artificial intelligence and how it will impact our world
- How COVID-19 may reshape the balance of power

Pearl of wisdom

'Learn from yesterday, live for today, hope for tomorrow.
The important thing is not to stop questioning.'

—Albert Einstein

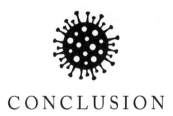

CONCLUSION

Hope for the Future

The world has been hijacked by fear and anxiety as a result of the COVID-19 pandemic and, with no end in sight of all the hype, hysteria and consequences surrounding it, many people are stressed to the limit. In the early stages of the disease, it appeared that an invisible monster had been let loose ready to pounce and claim its victims with reckless abandon. The monster, as we have seen, is not so much the disease itself, but the fear of it, together with the machinations of power that are keeping it alive and virile.

The scientific modelling that guided decision-making for medical and political leaders around the world has been wildly overestimated. The death toll, while tragic, has not been anywhere near as catastrophic as originally estimated. The tests are flawed, with many false positives and negatives. People assumed to have the disease are included in the case numbers. COVID-19 is recorded on the death certificate if someone dies of cancer and is diagnosed with this disease after the event.

Many people die with the disease and few from it. Only nine percent of all deaths can be contributed to COVID-19 alone and not compounded by other comorbidities. The average age of death from COVID-19 is 82.4 years, just slightly higher than deaths caused by other illnesses, with a median age of 81.5 years. Apply rounding and you end up with 82 years in both instances.

Cash-strapped hospitals are incentivised to treat COVID-19 patients, receiving $39,000 if they're placed on a ventilator. We hear so much about case numbers rising, but nothing about how death rates are falling. Hydroxychloroquine has proved to be a cheap, safe and effective treatment for COVID-19, especially when combined with zinc and azithromycin, but has been politically demonised and banned for public use based on corrupt science.

The race is on for a vaccine rollout. It will be highly profitable for billionaire patent owners as people demand salvation in a syringe, but will it be safe and effective? Orthomolecular medicine provides many safe and scientifically validated natural therapies that will prevent, improve or cure this disease, but such information has been censored from mainstream media. Free speech has gone out the window. Anyone not supporting the official narrative is shamed and their character slandered, including highly credentialed medical professionals.

The COVID-19 medical emergency was over for European countries in May or June 2020, but the political ramifications are still raging like an uncontrolled wildfire, supported largely by left-wing propaganda, according to Ivor Cummins. People dying from chronic diseases such as cancer, heart disease and stroke are now being re-classified as COVID deaths. Genevieve Briand, Assistant Director at Johns Hopkins University said, '… not only has COVID-19 had no effect on the percentage of deaths of older people, but it has also not increased the total number of deaths [from all causes]',[317] as discussed in chapter one. Socialism, communism, totalitarianism, whatever you like to call it, is on the rise and marching forward at an alarming rate. Is the fair go, fair share and fair say of democracy doomed?

Ever since March 2020, citizens of all nations worldwide have been bombarded with prophets of doom telling us that we are heading for a catastrophic fate by this widespread coronavirus pandemic. But just how much is fact and how much is fallacy largely depends on our beliefs and what prophet we wish to follow. 'Beware of false prophets, which come to you in sheep's clothing, but inwardly they are ravening wolves. You will recognise them by their fruits ...' (Matthew 7:15–20) English Standard Version.

It has been highlighted that politicians and health authorities can't be trusted, science is being suppressed for political and financial gain by the medical-political complex, and when this happens, people die. COVID-19 has unleashed corruption on a grand scale and powerful voices are advocating for more socialistic policies, wealth taxes and additional (draconian) regulations such as harder, more frequent lockdowns and the compulsory wearing of masks, even in the middle of nowhere. Now is the time for citizens to decide whether they want to embrace a dictatorship of communism or the liberty of democracy.

Historically, pandemics have been the instigator of major political and social reform. The COVID-19 pandemic can be a catalyst for a universal movement to disallow mass surveillance in any form. People can, for example, apply political pressure to insist on the implementation of

TEE technologies, returning all biometric data seized for surveillance and tracking to the owner for their own purposes in a secure and trusted environment on their mobile device. This will not only offer protection against software attacks such as identity theft and misuse of personal information but will also allow people to monitor their health and alert them to possible dangers in their vicinity.

Fear causes up to 90% of all disease, according to Dr Bruce Lipton; a sobering thought! But it can be disempowered by refusing to subscribe to it. By changing fearful thoughts into something more pleasant, such as writing a daily gratitude list, being grateful for what we *do* have in life, the energy frequency of the space-time continuum changes and miracles happen.

Taoist philosophy teaches us to be like water, 'Instead of resisting problems and adversity, try letting things be. Be like water and find ways to flow around obstacles with ease and grace.' Lao Tzu suggests we can learn a lot from water. While being one of the softest and most yielding substances, it's also one of the most powerful. Water can adapt to many forms—ice, liquid or steam, and become the shape of a glass, teapot or river. It also has the ability to cut through rock and move mountains. 'If we think about water flowing towards a rock, it will just flow around it. It doesn't get upset, it doesn't get angry, it doesn't get agitated. In fact, it doesn't feel much at all. When faced with an obstacle, somehow water finds a solution, without force, and without conflict.'

The purpose of this book is not for me to tell you what to think, but to allow you the freedom to think for yourself and decide what's best for you. We were all born to be free.

Free of the influence of power, corruption and greed. Free of political and medical tyranny and the social injustices that have plagued our world. Free to think for ourselves. May we all think wisely, resolve bravely, act kindly and live purely as we venture forth into the unknown. I wish you well on your journey and thank you for sharing part of mine.

---o◯o---

Your comments are welcome

I hope you found this book informative and helpful.
I value your feedback and would greatly appreciate it
if you would kindly leave a review at www.amazon.com
and/or www.goodreads.com. This will allow more readers
to become aware of the hidden truths outlined in this book
and potentially help them make informed decisions about
issues that may be important to them.

Many thanks
Margaret

ENDNOTES

1 Ivor Cummins, 'Viral Issue Crucial Update Sept 8th: The Science, Logic and Data Explained!', 8 September 2020, https://www.youtube.com/watch?v=8UvFhIFzaac

2 Dr Karina Reiss and Dr Sucharit Bhakdi, Corona False Alarm? Facts and Figures, Chelsea Green Publishing, London, UK (2020).

3 CDC, 'COVIDView Summary ending 5 December 2020', updated December 11, 2020, https://www.cdc.gov/coronavirus/2019-ncov/covid-data/covidview/past-reports/12112020.html

4 'Supplies – 506291-2020', TED Tenders Electronic Daily, 23 October 2020, https://ted.europa.eu/udl?uri=TED:NOTICE:506291-2020:TEXT:EN:HTML

5 Robert F. Kennedy, Jr., 'Robert F. Kennedy, Jr. Holds a Press Conference in Berlin After Launching CHD's Europe Charter', 28 August 2020, https://childrenshealthdefense.org/news/robert-f-kennedy-jr-holds-a-press-conference-in-berlin-after-launching-chds-europe-chapter/

6 Marise Payne, 'Morrison Government plans to set up taskforce to counter online disinformation', ABC News, 17 June 2020, https://www.abc.net.au/news/2020-06-17/foreign-minister-steps-up-criticism-china-global-cooperation/12362076

7 Peter Breggin, MD, COVID-19 & Public Health Totalitarianism: Untoward Effects on Individuals, Institutions and Society, 30 August 2020, https://breggin.com/coronavirus/NEW-COVID-19-LEGAL-REPORT.pdf

8 Vanessa Chalmers and Izzy Nikolic, 'Now UK will publish THREE separate Covid-19 death tolls amid statistics confusion after Public Health England fiasco which saw it count anyone who ever tested positive', Daily Mail Australia, 12 August 2020, https://www.dailymail.co.uk/news/article-8615723/Now-UK-publish-THREE-separate-Covid-19-death-tolls.html

9 World Health Organisation, 'International Guidelines for Certification and Classification (Coding) of COVID-19 as Cause of Death', 16 April 2020, https://www.who.int/classifications/icd/Guidelines_Cause_of_Death_COVID-19.pdf

10 Department of Health and Social Care, 'New UK-wide methodology agreed to record COVID-19 deaths'. 12 August 2020, https://www.gov.uk/government/news/new-uk-wide-methodology-agreed-to-record-covid-19-deaths

11 Marc Trabsky and Courtney Hempton, '"Died from' or 'died with' COVID-19? We need a transparent approach to counting coronavirus deaths', The Conversation, 9 September 2020, https://theconversation.com/died-from-or-died-with-covid-19-we-need-a-transparent-approach-to-counting-coronavirus-deaths-145438

12 Vanessa Chalmers and Izzy Nikolic, 'Now UK will publish THREE separate Covid-19 death tolls amid statistics confusion after Public Health England fiasco which saw it count anyone who ever tested positive', Daily Mail Australia, 12 August 2020, https://www.dailymail.co.uk/news/article-8615723/Now-UK-publish-THREE-separate-Covid-19-death-tolls.html

13 Tony Robbins, 'Where Focus Goes, Energy Flows: Create a vision for your business and your life', n/d, https://www.tonyrobbins.com/career-business/where-focus-goes-energy-flows/

14 John Mackenzie and David Smith, 'COVID-19: a novel zoonotic disease caused by a coronavirus from China: what we know and what we don't', Microbiology Australia, 17 March 2020, https://www.publish.csiro.au/ma/pdf/MA20013

15 Andrew Mark Miller, 'Imperial College Scientist who predicted 500K coronavirus deaths in UK adjusts figure to 20K or fewer', Washington Examiner, 30 March 2020, https://www.washingtonexaminer.com/news/imperial-college-scientist-who-predicted-500k-coronavirus-deaths-in-uk-revises-to-20k-or-less

16 John O'Sullivan, 'WHO Finally Admits COVID19 PCR Test Has A 'Problem'', Principia Scientific International, 17 December 2020, https://principia-scientific.com/who-finally-admits-covid19-pcr-test-has-a-problem/

17 Dr Joseph Mercola, 'Astonishing COVID-19 Testing Fraud Revealed', 13 January 2020, https://articles.mercola.com/sites/articles/archive/2021/01/13/coronavirus-pcr-testing.aspx

18 David DeGraw, et al., 'COVID Tests Scientifically Fraudulent, Epidemic of "False Positives"', 12 January 2021, https://www.globalresearch.ca/national-security-alert-covid-tests-scientifically-fraudulent-epidemic-false-positives/5720271

19 Lexy Hamilton-Smith, 'What is a false positive coronavirus test? How is it possible?' ABC News, 3 June 2020, https://www.abc.net.au/news/2020-06-03/coronavirus-queensland-how-is-a-false-posiitive-possible/12308076

20 Kit Knightly, 'WHO (finally) admits PCR tests create false positives', 18 December 2020, https://off-guardian.org/2020/12/18/who-finally-admits-pcr-tests-create-false-positives/

21 F. William Engdahl, 'Coronavirus Scandal Breaking in Merkel's Germany. False Positives and the Drosten PCR Test', 11 December 2020, https://www.globalresearch.ca/coronavirus-scandal-breaking-merkel-germany/5731891

22 Dr Pascale Sacre, 'The COVID-19 RT-PCR Test: How to Mislead Humanity. Using a "Test" to Lock Down Society', Global Research, 6 January 2021, https://willemfelderhof.com/the-covid-19-rt-pcr-test-how-to-mislead-all-humanity-using-a-test-to-lock-down-society/

23 Victor M. Corman, et al., 'Detection of 2019 novel coronavirus (2019-nCoV) by real-time RT-PCR', Eurosurveillance, January 2020, https://pubmed.ncbi.nlm.nih.gov/31992387/

24 F. William Engdahl, 'Coronavirus Scandal Breaking in Merkel's Germany. False Positives and the Drosten PCR Test', 11 December 2020, https://www.globalresearch.ca/coronavirus-scandal-breaking-merkel-germany/5731891

25 Kit Knightly, 'WHO (finally) admits PCR tests create false positives', 18 December 2020, https://off-guardian.org/2020/12/18/who-finally-admits-pcr-tests-create-false-positives/

26 Pieter Borger, PhD, et al., 'Review report Corman-Drosten et al. Eurosurveillance 2020', 27 November 2020, https://cormandrostenreview.com/report/

27 Rita Jaafar, et al., 'Correlation Between 3790 Quantitative Polymerase Chain Reaction—Positives Samples and Positive Cell Cultures, Including 1941 Severe Acute Respiratory Syndrome Coronavirus 2 Isolates', Clinical Infectious Diseases, 28 September 2020, https://academic.oup.com/cid/advance-article/doi/10.1093/cid/ciaa1491/5912603

28 F. William Engdahl, 'Coronavirus Scandal Breaking in Merkel's Germany. False Positives and the Drosten PCR Test', 11 December 2020, https://www.globalresearch.ca/coronavirus-scandal-breaking-merkel-germany/5731891

29 Dr Joseph Mercola, 'Astonishing COVID-19 Testing Fraud Revealed', 13 January 2020, https://articles.mercola.com/sites/articles/archive/2021/01/13/coronavirus-pcr-testing.aspx

30 Jim Grisanzio interview with Dr Fauci (Twitter video), 12 November 2020, https://twitter.com/jimgris/status/1326518250386063361

31 John O'Sullivan, 'WHO Finally Admits COVID19 PCR Test Has A 'Problem'', Principia Scientific International, 17 December 2020, https://principia-scientific.com/who-finally-admits-covid19-pcr-test-has-a-problem/

32 Kit Knightly, 'WHO (finally) admits PCR tests create false positives', 18 December 2020, https://off-guardian.org/2020/12/18/who-finally-admits-pcr-tests-create-false-positives/

33 Jim Grisanzio interview with Dr Fauci (Twitter video), 12 November 2020, https://twitter.com/jimgris/status/1326518250386063361

34 Donald L Luskin, 'The Failed Experiment of Covid Lockdowns: New data suggests that social distancing and re-opening haven't determined the spread', The Wall Street Journal, Opinion, 1 September 2020, https://www.wsj.com/articles/the-failed-experiment-of-covid-lockdowns-11599000890

35 Rabail Chaudhry, et al., 'A country level analysis measuring the impact of government actions, country preparedness and socioeconomic factors on COVID-19 mortality and related health outcomes', The Lancet, 21 July 2020, https://www.thelancet.com/journals/eclinm/article/PIIS2589-5370(20)30208-X/fulltext

36 Simon N Wood, 'Did COVID-19 infections decline before UK lockdown?' University of Edinburgh, 21 September 2020, https://arxiv.org/pdf/2005.02090.pdf

37 Paul R Hunter, et al., 'Impact of non-pharmaceutical interventions against COVID-19 in Europe: a quasi-experimental study', Research Gate preprint, 6 May 2020, https://www.researchgate.net/publication/341199560_Impact_of_non-pharmaceutical_interventions_against_COVID-19_in_Europe_a_quasi-experimental_study

38 Sunetra Gupta, Professor, 'Long periods of lockdown could weaken the immune system and leave people more vulnerable to dangerous viruses, Oxford epidemiologist warns', Daily Mail Australia, 28 June 2020, https://www.dailymail.co.uk/news/article-8466931/Lockdown-leave-people-vulnerable-dangerous-viruses-Oxford-epidemiologist-warns.html

39 Ian Hickie, Professor, 'The silent death toll of COVID-19 revealed: Huge 25 per cent jump in suicides each year', 25 July 2020, https://www.news.com.au/lifestyle/health/health-problems/the-silent-death-toll-of-covid19-revealed-huge-25-per-cent-jump-in-suicides-each-year/news-story/b4154626a16c9cc25c3b79b7880041ef

40 Michael Doyle, 'WHO doctor says lockdowns should not be main coronavirus defence', ABC News, 12 October 2020, https://www.abc.net.au/news/2020-10-12/world-health-organization-coronavirus-lockdown-advice/12753688

41 David Nabarro, M.D., 'Reflections about the middle path', n/d, https://www.4sd.info/covid-19-narratives/reflections-about-the-middle-path/

42 Peter Lewis, 'What was the deadliest weapon in World War II? Starvation, which killed 20 million people', Mail Online, 28 January 2011, https://www.dailymail.co.uk/home/books/article-1351152/Q-What-deadliest-weapon-World-War-II-A-Starvation-killed-20-million-people-THE-TASTE-OF-WAR-BY-LIZZIE-COLLINGHAM.html

43 Stephen Robinson, 'Remembering the war in New Guinea—What did the soldiers eat?' 1 June 2004, http://ajrp.awm.gov.au/ajrp/remember.nsf/pages/NT000017BA

44 Centers for Disease Control and Prevention, 'Interim Clinical Guidance for Management of Patients with Confirmed Coronavirus Disease (COVID-19)', 30 June 2020, https://stacks.cdc.gov/view/cdc/89980

45 Hans K Biesalski, 'Vitamin D deficiency and co-morbidities in COVID-19 patients—A fatal relationship?' Nutrition and Food Science Journal, 25 June 2020, https://www.researchgate.net/publication/341995638_Vitamin_D_deficiency_and_co-morbidities_in_COVID-19_patients_-_A_fatal_relationship

46 Robert Verity, PhD, et al., 'Estimates of the severity of coronavirus disease 2019: a model-based analysis', The Lancet, 30 March 2020, https://www.thelancet.com/journals/laninf/article/PIIS1473-3099(20)30243-7/fulltext

47 Australian Government Department of Health, 'COVID-19 Australia: Epidemiology Report 22', 2 August 2020, https://doi.org/10.33321/cdi.2020.44.69

48 World Health Organisation, 'International Guidelines for Certification and Classification (Coding) of COVID-19 as Cause of Death', 16 April 2020, https://www.who.int/classifications/icd/Guidelines_Cause_of_Death_COVID-19.pdf

49 Katie Pavlich, 'The Way the US is Counting Wuhan Coronavirus Deaths Seems Problematic', 8 April 2020, https://townhall.com/tipsheet/katiepavlich/2020/04/08/the-way-the-us-is-counting-wuhan-coronavirus-deaths-seems-problematic-n2566543

50 Anthony S. Fauci, M.D., et al., 'COVID-19—Navigating the Uncharted', The New England Journal of Medicine, 28 February 2020, https://www.nejm.org/doi/full/10.1056/NEJMe2002387

51 World Health Organisation, 'WHO Director-General's remarks at a media briefing on COVID-19 outbreak on 17 February 2020', 17 February 2020, https://www.who.int/director-general/speeches/detail/who-director-general-s-remarks-at-the-media-briefing-on-covid-2019-outbreak-on-17-february-2020

52 Ronald Bailey, 'What Percentage of COVID-19 Patients Are Likely to Die?' 3 April 2020, https://reason.com/2020/04/03/what-percentage-of-covid-19-patients-are-likely-to-die/

53 The Johns Hopkins News-Letter, 'A closer look at U.S. deaths due to COVID-19', 22 November 2020, https://corona-transition.org/IMG/pdf/a_closer_look_at_u.s._deaths_due_to_covid-19_-_the_johns_hopkins_news-letter.pdf

54 Stephen Lendman, 'The Great 2020 Seasonal Flu/Influenza Disappearing Act', 31 December 2020, https://stephenlendman.org/2020/12/the-great-2020-seasonal-flu-influenza-disappearing-act/

55 Jiji Kyodo, 'Japan study finds 98% of COVID-19 patients had immunity six months later', The Japan Times, 3 December 2020, https://www.japantimes.co.jp/news/2020/12/03/national/coronavirus-immunity-study/

56 Andrew T. Levin, et al., 'Assessing the Age Specificity of Infection Fatality Rates for COVID-19: Systemic Review, Meta-Analysis, and Public Policy Implications', European Journal of Epidemiology, 10 November 2020, https://doi.org/10.1007/s10654-020-00698-1

57 Kaya Burgess, 'Average Age of coronavirus fatalities is 82', The Times, 10 October 2020, https://www.thetimes.co.uk/article/average-age-of-coronavirus-fatalities-is-82-pcwqrzdzz

58 Nicoletta Lanese, 'The CDC is lumping COVID-19 viral and antibody tests together. Here's why that's bad', 21 May 2020, https://www.livescience.com/cdc-combined-covid-19-diagnostic-and-antibody-tests.html

59 Centers for Disease Control and Prevention, 'Test for Past Infection', 29 October 2020, https://www.cdc.gov/coronavirus/2019-ncov/testing/serology-overview.html

60 Centers for Disease Control and Prevention, 'Coronavirus Disease 2019 (COVID-19) 2020 Interim Case Definition, Approved August 5 2020', https://wwwn.cdc.gov/nndss/conditions/coronavirus-disease-2019-covid-19/case-definition/2020/08/05/

61 Malcolm Kendrick, M.D., 'COVID–why terminology really, really matters', 4 September 2020, https://drmalcolmkendrick.org/2020/09/04/covid-why-terminology-really-matters/

62 Rich Condit, Professor, 'Infection Fatality Rate—A Critical Missing Piece for Managing COVID-19', 5 April 2020, https://www.virology.ws/2020/04/05/infection-fatality-rate-a-critical-missing-piece-for-managing-covid-19/

63 Kate Ng, 'Tanzania coronavirus kits raise suspicion after goat and pawpaw test positive', 12 May 2020, https://www.independent.co.uk/news/world/africa/coronavirus-tanzania-test-kits-suspicion-goat-pawpaw-positive-a9501291.html

64 The New Daily ,'I tested positive for COVID-19, but that was the least of my worries', 31 May 2020, https://thenewdaily.com.au/news/national/2020/05/30/coronavirus-test-debacle/

65 C Raina MacIntyre, et al., 'A cluster randomised trial of cloth masks compared with medical masks in healthcare workers', British Medical Journal, 22 April 2015, https://bmjopen.bmj.com/content/bmjopen/5/4/e006577.full.pdf

66 John T Brooks, M.D., et al., 'Universal Masking to Prevent SARS-CoV-2 Transmission—The Time Is Now', Journal of the American Medical Association (JAMA), 14 July 2020, https://jamanetwork.com/journals/jama/fullarticle/2768532

67 Encyclopaedia Britannica, 'Coronavirus', 27 August 2020, https://www.britannica.com/science/coronavirus-virus-group

68 Michael Mosley, M.D., COVID-19: What you need to know about the coronavirus and the race for a vaccine, Simon & Schuster (Australia) Pty Ltd, 2020.

69 Queensland University of Technology, 'New mask material can remove virus-size nanoparticles', 16 April 2020, https://www.qut.edu.au/institute-for-future-environments/about/news?id=161592

70 World Health Organisation, 'Historic health assembly ends with global commitment to COVID-19 response', 19 May 2020, https://www.who.int/news/item/19-05-2020-historic-health-assembly-ends-with-global-commitment-to-covid-19-response

71 Daniel Hurst, 'Australia hails global support for independent coronavirus investigation', The Guardian Australia, 18 May 2020, https://www.theguardian.com/world/2020/may/18/australia-wins-international-support-for-independent-coronavirus-inquiry

72 Bernard Lagan, 'Lobster left to rot as China blocks Australian trade', 3 November 2020, The Times, https://www.thetimes.co.uk/article/lobster-left-to-rot-as-china-blocks-australian-trade-xt5kdxrdg

73 Dannielle Maguire, 'What we know about the 'sophisticated, state-based' cyber attack on Australia', 19 June 2020, https://www.abc.net.au/news/2020-06-19/cyber-attack-no-australian-government-organisations-explained/12373190

74 World Health Organisation, 'WHO Director-General opening remarks at the Member State Briefing on the COVID-19 pandemic evaluation – 9 July 2020', 9 July 2020, https://www.who.int/director-general/speeches/detail/who-director-general-opening-remarks-at-the-member-state-briefing-on-the-covid-19-pandemic-evaluation---9-july-2020

75 Christopher Klein, 'China Epicenter of 1918 Flu Pandemic, Historian Says', 7 March 2019, https://www.history.com/news/china-epicenter-of-1918-flu-pandemic-historian-says

76 Sharri Markson, 'Chinese scientists linked to virus probe worked in Australia', The Daily Telegraph, 28 April 2020, https://senatorpaterson.com.au/2020/04/28/chinese-scientists-linked-to-virus-probe-worked-in-australia/

77 Stephanie Hegarty, 'The Chinese doctor who tried to warn others about coronavirus', BBC News, 6 February 2020, https://www.bbc.com/news/world-asia-china-51364382

78 Gordon Corera, 'Coronavirus: China rejects call for probe into origins of disease', BBC News, 24 April 2020, https://www.bbc.com/news/world-asia-china-52420536

79 Kamran Abbasi, 'COVID-19: Politicisation, "corruption," and suppression of science', British Medical Journal, 13 November 2020, https://www.bmj.com/content/371/bmj.m4425

80 Eric Worrall, 'What is the Great Reset?' 21 November 2020, https://wattsupwiththat.com/2020/11/21/what-is-the-great-reset/

81 Colin Todhunter, 'Dystopian "Great Reset": "Own Nothing and Be Happy", Being Human in 2030', Global Research, 9 November 2020, https://www.globalresearch.ca/own-nothing-happy-being-human-2030/5728960

82 Joseph Mercola, M.D., 'Who Pressed the Great Reset Button?' 20 November 2020, https://wakeup-world.com/2020/11/20/who-pressed-the-great-reset-button/

83 Ray DiLorenzo, 'The Great Reset: What You Need to Know', Canada Free Press, 24 November 2020, https://canadafreepress.com/article-ng/the-great-reset-what-you-need-to-know

84 Justin Haskins, 'Introducing the 'Great Reset,' world leaders' radical plan to transform the economy', 25 June 2020, https://thehill.com/opinion/energy-environment/504499-introducing-the-great-reset-world-leaders-radical-plan-to

85 Will Feuer and Noah Higgins-Dunn, 'Asymptomatic spread of coronavirus is 'very rare,' WHO says', 8 June 2020, https://www.cnbc.com/2020/06/08/asymptomatic-coronavirus-patients-arent-spreading-new-infections-who-says.html

86 Berkely Lovelace Jr., Jasmine Kim, Will Feuer, 'WHO walks back comments on asymptomatic coronavirus spread, says much is still unknown', 9 June 2020, https://www.cnbc.com/2020/06/09/who-scrambles-to-clarify-comments-on-asymptomatic-coronavirus-spread-much-is-still-unknown.html

87 Ming Gao, et al., 'A Study on Infectivity of Asymptomatic SARS-CoV-2 Carriers', Journal of Respiratory Medicine, 13 May 2020, https://pubmed.ncbi.nlm.nih.gov/32513410/

88 Shiyi Cao, et al., ' Post-lockdown SARS-CoV-2 nucleic acid screening in nearly ten million residents of Wuhan, China', Nature Communications, November 2020, https://pubmed.ncbi.nlm.nih.gov/33219229/

89 Americans for Tax Fairness, 'Net worth of U.S. Billionaires has soared by $1 trillion—to total of $4 trillion—since pandemic began', 8 December 2020, https://americansfortaxfairness.org/issue/net-worth-u-s-billionaires-soared-1-trillion-total-4-trillion-since-pandemic-began/

90 World Health Organisation, 'A World at Risk: Annual report on global preparedness for health emergencies', Global Preparedness Monitoring Board, September 2019, https://apps.who.int/gpmb/assets/annual_report/GPMB_annualreport_2019.pdf

91 Infectious Disease News, 'Trump warned about inevitable infectious disease outbreak', 16 February 2017, https://www.healio.com/news/infectious-disease/20170208/trump-warned-about-inevitable-infectious-disease-outbreak

92 Corazon Miller, 'Bill Gates predicted a coronavirus-like outbreak – down to it starting at a Chinese market – in 2019 Netflix documentary show 'The Next Pandemic", 1 February 2020, https://www.dailymail.co.uk/news/article-7951293/Bill-Gates-Predicted-Coronavirus-Like-Outbreak-2019-Netflix-Documentary.html

93 'Bioterrorism: "… be ready for pandemic two! I call this pandemic one." Bill Gates 24 April 2020', 28 April 2020, https://www.youtube.com/watch?v=g_NEe0eHgfY

94 Sangetta Nair, 'UK's new mutated coronavirus strain highly infectious: UK PM orders lockdown, India suspends UK flights', 21 December 2020, https://www.jagranjosh.com/current-affairs/uk-new-mutated-coronavirus-strain-highly-infectious-tier4-covid19-rules-announced-in-london-get-details-here-1608542669-1

95 'DOD study raises tantalizing question: does flu shot increase vulnerability to coronavirus?' 3 June 2020, https://justthenews.com/politics-policy/coronavirus/does-influenza-vaccine-have-any-effect-other-viruses

96 Coronavirus News, 'Science backs Dr. Judy Mikovits' warning that COVID vaccine could kill 50 Million Americans', 19 November 2020, https://coronanews123.wordpress.com/2020/11/19/dr-judy-mikovits-claims-of-50-million-americans-dead-of-covid-vaccine-not-unsubstantiated/

97 Australian government, 'Australia and the world in the time of COVID-19', 16 June 2020, https://www.foreignminister.gov.au/minister/marise-payne/speech/australia-and-world-time-covid-19

98 Clive Hamilton & Mareike Ohlberg, Hidden Hand: Exposing How the Chinese Communist Party is Reshaping the World, Hardie Grant Publishing, Victoria, Australia, 2020.

99 Stephen Dziedzic and Melissa Clarke, 'Morrison Government plans to set up taskforce to counter online disinformation', ABC News, 17 June 2020, https://www.abc.net.au/news/2020-06-17/foreign-minister-steps-up-criticism-china-global-cooperation/12362076

100 Eddy Rodriguez, 'China Donates $30 Million to World Health Organisation in Show of 'Support' After Trump Pulls Funding', 23 April 2020, https://www.newsweek.com/china-donates-30-million-world-health-organization-show-support-after-trump-pulls-funding-1499854

101 Javier C Hernandez, 'Trump slammed the WHO over coronavirus. He's not alone.', Chicago Tribune, 8 April 2020, https://www.chicagotribune.com/coronavirus/sns-nyt-world-leaders-questions-who-response-20200408-mampsbgo2zbujpyvazbdsvij7q-story.html

102 Michael J. Imperiale and Arturo Casadevall, 'A New Approach to Evaluating the Risk-Benefit Equation for Dual-Use and Gain-of-Function Research of Concern', Frontiers in Bioengineering and Biotechnology, 8 March 2020, https://www.frontiersin.org/articles/10.3389/fbioe.2018.00021/full

103 Michael Selgelid, in 'Gain-Of-Function Research: Ethical Analysis', Science and Engineering Ethics, 8 August 2020, https://pubmed.ncbi.nlm.nih.gov/27502512/

104 US Department of Health and Human Services, 'Gain-of-Function Research', 6 March 2019, https://www.phe.gov/s3/dualuse/Pages/GainOfFunction.aspx

105 Lynn Klotz, 'Human error in high-biocontainment labs: a likely pandemic threat', 25 February 2019, https://thebulletin.org/2019/02/human-error-in-high-biocontainment-labs-a-likely-pandemic-threat/

106 Wuze Ren, et al., 'Difference in Receptor Usage between Severe Acute Respiratory Syndrome (SARS) Coronavirus and SARS-Like Coronavirus of Bat Origin', Journal of Virology, February 2008, https://www.ncbi.nlm.nih.gov/pmc/articles/PMC2258702/

107 Tobias Hoonhout, 'U.S. Diplomats Warned about Safety Risks in Wuhan Labs Studying Bats Two Years before Coronavirus Outbreak', 14 April 2020, https://www.nationalreview.com/news/u-s-diplomats-warned-about-safety-risks-in-wuhan-labs-studying-bats-two-years-before-coronavirus-outbreak/

108 The Science Times, 'UK Fears Coronavirus Might Have Actually Been Leaked from a China Lab', 6 April 2020, https://www.sciencetimes.com/articles/25214/20200406/uk-fears-coronavirus-actually-leaked-china-lab.htm

109 Jim Hayek, "China Blamed Wet Market To 'Deflect Blame' From Lab, DESTROYED Evidence, Fox News Reports', 16 April 2020, https://americantruthtoday.com/politics/2020/04/16/china-blamed-wet-market-to-deflect-blame-from-lab-destroyed-evidence-fox-news-reports/

110 Gordon G. Chang, 'Gordon G. Chang: China falsely blames US for coronavirus pandemic', Fox News, 12 March 2020, https://www.foxnews.com/opinion/gordon-g-chang-china-falsely-blames-us-for-coronavirus-pandemic

111 Erin Olszewski, 'Perspectives on the Pandemic, episode nine, 'The (Undercover) Epicentre Nurse', n/d, https://www.brighteon.com/034c2c49-0053-44ab-9a8a-0f8816a1c211

112 'COVID-19 was created in the Wuhan laboratory: Professor Giuseppe Tritto', 25 September 2020, https://www.wionews.com/world/covid-19-was-created-in-the-wuhan-laboratory-professor-giuseppe-tritto-330053

113 Joseph Mercola, M.D., 'More Experts Point to SARS-CoV-2 Being Created in a Lab', 4 September 2020, https://www.organicconsumers.org/news/more-experts-point-sars-cov-2-being-lab-created

114 Corporate Crime Reporter, 'Andrew Kimbrell on the Origins of COVID-19', 11 August 2020, https://www.corporatecrimereporter.com/news/200/andrew-kimbrell-on-the-origins-of-covid-19/

115 Stephen Johnson, 'Health boss weighs in on theory COVID-19 originated in a Wuhan lab and doubles down on Australia's call for independent inquiry that has sparked trade threats from China', Daily Mail, 25 May 2020, https://www.dailymail.co.uk/news/article-8353801/Health-Minister-Greg-Hunt-addresses-Mail-Sunday-revelation-COVID-19-originated-lab.html

116 Judy Mikovits, PhD, Joseph Mercola, M.D., 'SARS-CoV-2-Interview with Judy Mikovits', 4 May 2020, https://www.youtube.com/watch?v=eSgN8ONNKVs. Transcript, 'Is SARS-Co-V-2 a Manufactured Virus? A Special Interview with Judy Mikovits', http://totuusrokotteista.fi/v3/files/T428Ng1czD/ttav+Interview-JudyMikovits-IsSARSCoV2aManufacturedVirus.pdf

117 Erin Olszewski, 'Perspectives on the pandemic: the (undercover) epicentre nurse', 9 June 2020, https://www.youtube.com/watch?v=UIDsKdeFOmQ

118 Stacey Lennox, 'New Data from the CDC Shows 6% of Deaths Are Due to COVID-19 Alone', 31 August 2020, https://pjmedia.com/news-and-politics/stacey-lennox/2020/08/31/new-data-from-the-cdc-shows-6-of-deaths-are-due-to-covid-19-alone-n867807

119 Office of the High Commissioner for Human Rights (OHCHR), 'COVID-19: Exceptional measures should not be cover for human rights abuses and violations – Bachelet', 27 April 2020, https://www.ohchr.org/EN/NewsEvents/Pages/DisplayNews.aspx?NewsID=25828&LangID=E

120 Antonio Guterrs, 'We are all in this Together: Human Rights and COVID-19 Response and Recovery', United Nations, 23 April 2020, https://www.un.org/en/un-coronavirus-communications-team/we-are-all-together-human-rights-and-covid-19-response-and

121 Keith Scott-Mumby, Professor, 'The New Abnormal', 6 August 2020, https://drkeithsown.myshopify.com/blogs/alternative-doctor/the-new-abnormal

122 United Nations, 'COVID-19 and Human Rights: Human rights are critical – for the response and recovery', April 2020, https://unsdg.un.org/sites/default/files/2020-04/COVID-19-and-Human-Rights.pdf

123 Eva Valera, PhD, 'When lockdown is not actually safer: Intimate partner violence during COVID-19', Harvard Health Publishing: Harvard Medical School, 7 July 2020, https://www.health.harvard.edu/blog/when-lockdown-is-not-actually-safer-intimate-partner-violence-during-covid-19-2020070720529

124 Joseph Mercola, M.D., 'Why Lockdowns Don't Work and Hurt the Most Vulnerable', 30 December 2020, https://articles.mercola.com/sites/articles/archive/2020/12/30/lockdowns-do-not-work.aspx

125 Yellowlees Douglass, PhD, 'The Costs of Social Isolation: Loneliness and COVID-19', 29 April 2020, https://www.psychiatryadvisor.com/home/topics/general-psychiatry/costs-of-social-isolation-loneliness-covid19/

126 Jo-An Atkinson, A/Professor, et al., 'Road to Recovery: Restoring Australia's Mental Wealth', University of Sydney, 27 July 2020, https://apo.org.au/sites/default/files/resource-files/2020-08/apo-nid307435.pdf

127 Dr Agomoni Ganguli Mitra, 'Social justice may be our greatest antidote', 6 April 2020, https://www.ed.ac.uk/covid-19-response/expert-insights/social-justice-in-a-time-of-pandemic

128 Kelly Burke, 'US Coronavirus patients placed on ventilators have grim prognosis, study finds', 27 April 2020, https://7news.com.au/lifestyle/health-wellbeing/us-coronavirus-patients-placed-on-ventilators-have-grim-prognosis-study-finds-c-996937

129 Robert Langreth, 'New Study Shows Nearly 9 in 10 Covid-19 Patients on Ventilators Don't Make It', 23 April 2020, https://www.bloomberg.com/news/articles/2020-04-22/almost-9-in-10-covid-19-patients-on-ventilators-died-in-study

130 National Research Council Canada, 'The National Research Council of Canada and CanSino Biologics Inc. announce collaboration to advance vaccine against COVID-19', 12 May 2020, https://www.canada.ca/en/national-research-council/news/2020/05/the-national-research-council-of-canada-and-cansino-biologics-inc-announce-collaboration-to-advance-vaccine-against-covid-19.html

131 Jonathan Abbamonte, 'Which COVID-19 vaccines will be derived from aborted children's cell lines?' 11 June 2020, https://www.lifesitenews.com/opinion/which-covid-19-vaccines-will-be-derived-from-aborted-childrens-cell-lines

132 CDC, 'Vaccine Excipient and Media Summary', March 2018, https://vaccine.guide/vaccine-ingredients/overview/cdc-vaccine-excipient-and-media-summary/

133 Corvelva, 'Vaccinegate: MRC-5 contained in Priorix Tetra – Complete genome sequencing', 27 September 2019, https://childrenshealthdefense.org/wp-content/uploads/CORVELVA-MRC-5-contained-in-Priorix-Tetra-Complete-genome-sequencing.pdf

134 British Medical Journal, 'The Nuremberg Code (1947)', 7 December 1996, https://media.tghn.org/medialibrary/2011/04/BMJ_No_7070_Volume_313_The_Nuremberg_Code.pdf

135 Bridget Haire, et al., 'Raising Rates of Childhood Vaccination: The Trade-off Between Coercion and Trust', Journal of Bioethical Inquiry, 1 March 2018, https://link.springer.com/article/10.1007/s11673-018-9841-1

136 Cheryl K. Chumley, 'Coronavirus hype biggest political hoax in history', 28 April 2020, https://www.washingtontimes.com/news/2020/apr/28/coronavirus-hype-biggest-political-hoax-in-history/

137 Joseph Mercola, M.D., 'New Report Claims to Shed Light on SARS-CoV-2 Origin', 27 September 2020, https://articles.mercola.com/sites/articles/archive/2020/09/27/chinese-whistleblower-coronavirus.aspx

138 Ana Rivas, et al., article 'Covid-19 Vaccines: What's Coming and When?' The Wall Street Journal, 22 December 2020, https://www.wsj.com/articles/covid-19-vaccines-whats-coming-and-when-11598882964

139 Amy McKeever, 'Here's the Latest on COVID-19 Vaccines', 23 November 2020, https://yalibnan.com/2020/11/23/heres-the-latest-on-covid-19-vaccines/

140 Nick Triggle, 'Covid-19 vaccine: First person receives Pfizer jab in UK', 8 December 2020, https://www.bbc.com/news/uk-55227325

141 The New Daily, 'FDA publishes first peer-reviewed report on Pfizer trial as Britain rolls out COVID vaccine', 15 December 2020, https://thenewdaily.com.au/news/coronavirus/2020/12/09/pfizer-oxford-astrazeneca-vaccines/

142 Aljazeera, 'People with anaphylaxis history should not take Pfizer COVID shot', 10 December 2020, https://www.aljazeera.com/news/2020/12/10/people-with-anaphylaxis-history-should-not-take-pfizer-covid-shot

143 Niran Al-Agba, M.D., 'Here's what Pfizer's COVID vaccine does to combat the virus', 9 December 2020, https://www.kitsapsun.com/story/opinion/columnists/2020/12/09/heres-what-covid-vaccine-does-combat-virus/6492657002/

144 The University of Alberta Faculty of Medicine & Dentistry, 'ACE2 protein protects against severe COVID-19: Study', 10 December 2020, https://medicalxpress.com/news/2020-12-ace2-protein-severe-covid-.html

145 Michael Mosley, M.D., COVID-19: What you need to know about the coronavirus and the race for a vaccine, Simon & Schuster (Australia) Pty Ltd, 2020.

146 Ross Walter, 'Busted! COVID vaccine manufacturers committed fraud on their vaccine trials', 4 December 2020, http://www.rosswalter.com.au/articles/december-04th-20203799345

147 Niran Al-Agba, M.D., 'Here's what Pfizer's COVID vaccine does to combat the virus', 9 December 2020, https://www.kitsapsun.com/story/opinion/columnists/2020/12/09/heres-what-covid-vaccine-does-combat-virus/6492657002/

148 Dr Joseph Mercola, 'Side Effects and Data Gaps Raise Questions on COVID vaccine', 26 January 2021, https://articles.mercola.com/sites/articles/archive/2021/01/26/covid-vaccine-side-effects.aspx

149 Peter Doshi, 'Peter Doshi: Pfizer and Moderna's "95% effective" vaccines—let's be cautious and see the full data', The British Medical Journal Opinion, 26 November 2020, https://blogs.bmj.com/bmj/2020/11/26/peter-doshi-pfizer-and-modernas-95-effective-vaccines-lets-be-cautious-and-first-see-the-full-data/

150 Nick Pearson, 'Australia will not automatically approve Pfizer vaccine in wake of UK, US rollout', 11 December 2020, https://www.9news.com.au/national/coronavirus-australia-pfizer-vaccine-not-automatically-approved-based-on-uk-us/69f12145-4a3d-462f-acba-6c58d9f4676f

151 Marie Dubert, et al., In 'Case report study of the first five COVID-19 patients treated with remdesivir in France', 26 June 2020, https://www.sciencedirect.com/science/article/pii/S1201971220305282

152 Kate Aubusson and Ashleigh McMillan, 'New drug to help Australian patients fight off COVID-19 comes with 'Caveats'', The Sydney Morning Herald, 11 July 2020, https://www.smh.com.au/national/new-drug-to-help-australian-patients-fight-off-covid-19-comes-with-caveats-20200711-p55b67.html

153 Yeming Want, M.D., et al., 'Remdesivir in adults with severe COVID-19: a randomised, double-blind, placebo-controlled, multicentre trial', The Lancet, 29 April 2020, https://www.thelancet.com/journals/lancet/article/PIIS0140-6736(20)31022-9/fulltext

154 Hugh Cassiere, M.D. and Mikaela Wolf, ''There is light at the end of the tunnel': New York Health care workers share lessons from COVID-19 frontlines', 31 July 2020, https://news.yahoo.com/light-end-tunnel-york-health-134645356.html

155 ABC News, 'Remdesivir approved by the Therapeutic Goods Administration for severe coronavirus cases', 11 July 2020, https://www.abc.net.au/news/2020-07-11/remdesivir-approved-by-tga-coronavirus-covid-19-australia/12446036

156 Kate Aubusson and Ashleigh McMillan, 'New drug to help Australian patients fight off COVID-19 comes with 'Caveats'', The Sydney Morning Herald, 11 July 2020, https://www.smh.com.au/national/new-drug-to-help-australian-patients-fight-off-covid-19-comes-with-caveats-20200711-p55b67.html

157 Fadela Chaib, 'WHO welcomes preliminary results about dexamethasone use in treating critically ill COVID-19 patients', World Health Organisation news release, 16 June 2020, https://www.who.int/news/item/16-06-2020-who-welcomes-preliminary-results-about-dexamethasone-use-in-treating-critically-ill-covid-19-patients

158 National Institutes of Health (NIH), 'Chloroquine or Hydroxychloroquine With or Without Azithromycin', 9 October 2020, https://www.covid19treatmentguidelines.nih.gov/antiviral-therapy/chloroquine-or-hydroxychloroquine-with-or-without-azithromycin/

159 National Institutes of Health (NIH), 'NIH halts clinical trial of hydroxychloroquine', 20 June 2020, https://www.nih.gov/news-events/news-releases/nih-halts-clinical-trial-hydroxychloroquine

160 National Institutes of Health (NIH), 'Chloroquine or Hydroxychloroquine With or Without Azithromycin', updated 9 October 2020, https://www.covid19treatmentguidelines.nih.gov/antiviral-therapy/chloroquine-or-hydroxychloroquine-with-or-without-azithromycin/

161 Martin J Vincent, et al., 'Chloroquine is a potent inhibitor of SARS coronavirus infection and spread', Virology Journal, 22 August 2005, https://pubmed.ncbi.nlm.nih.gov/16115318/

162 Huihui Wang, et al., 'The genetic sequence, origin, and diagnosis of SARS-CoV-2', European Journal of Clinical Microbiology and Infectious Diseases, 24 April 2020, https://pubmed.ncbi.nlm.nih.gov/32333222/

163 Rep. Ron Paul and Prof. Michel Chossudovsky, 'Anthony Fauci is Out, "Sidelined" by Trump. Enter Dr. Scott Atlas to the Coronavirus Task Force', 17 August 2020, https://www.globalresearch.ca/fauci-out-common-sense-returning/5721406

164 Kiran Stacey and Hannah Kuchler, 'Jeff Zients, the 'Mr. Fix It' Biden put in charge of tackling the COVID-19 crisis', Los Angeles Times, 20 January 2021, https://www.latimes.com/world-nation/story/2021-01-20/joe-biden-jeff-zients-covid-19-crisis

165 Yoni Kempinski, 'Dr. Zelenko promises: Use of hydroxychloroquine with zinc 'will end coronavirus plague", 22 May 2020, https://www.israelnationalnews.com/News/News.aspx/280690

166 Samia Arshad, et al., 'Treatment with hydroxychloroquine, azithromycin, and combination in patients hospitalised with COVID-19', International Journal of Infectious Diseases, 29 June 2020, https://www.ijidonline.com/action/showPdf?pii=S1201-9712%2820%2930534-8

167 Sharyl Attkisson, 'BREAKING: Hydroxychloroquine lowers Covid-19 death rate, study finds', 2 July 2020, https://sharylattkisson.com/2020/07/breaking-hydroxychloroquine-lowers-covid-19-death-rate-study-finds/

168 Anne Flaherty and Jordyn Phelps, 'Fauci throws cold water on Trump's declaration that malaria drug chloroquine is a 'game changer", ABC News, 21 March 2020, https://abcnews.go.com/Politics/fauci-throws-cold-water-trumps-declaration-malaria-drug/story?id=69716324

169 Mandeep R Mehra, et al., 'Hydroxychloroquine or chloroquine with or without a macrolide for treatment of COVID-19: a multinational registry analysis', The Lancet, 22 May 2020, https://covid19criticalcare.com/wp-content/uploads/2020/05/HCQ-decreased-in-hospital-survival.pdf

170 Pierre Kory, M.D., '"I Can't Keep Doing This": Doctor pleads for review of data during COVID-19 Senate hearing', 8 December 2020, https://www.youtube.com/watch?v=Tq8SXOBy-4w

171 Dee McLachlan, 'Pierre Kory, M.D — Ivermectin has "Miraculous Impact", It "Obliterates" Covid-19', 13 December 2020, https://gumshoenews. com/2020/12/13/pierre-kory-m-d-ivermectin-has-miraculous-impact-it-obliterates-covid-19/

172 Pierre Kory, M.D. et al., 'Review of the Emerging Evidence Demonstrating the Efficacy of Ivermectin in the Prophylaxis and Treatment of COVID-19', Preprint, 13 November 2020, https://osf.io/wx3zn/

173 Erwan Sallard, et al., 'Type I interferons as a potential treatment against COVID-19', 7 April 2020, https://www.ncbi.nlm.nih.gov/pmc/articles/PMC7138382/

174 Judy Mikovits, M.D. and Joseph Mercola, M.D., 'SARS-CoV-2-Interview with Judy Mikovits', 4 May 2020, https://www.youtube.com/watch?v=eSgN8ONNKVs

175 Ruben Manuel Luciano Colunga Biancatelli, et at., 'Quercetin and Vitamin C: An Experimental, Synergistic Therapy for the Prevention and Treatment of SARS-CoV-2 Related Disease (COVID-19)', Frontiers in Immunology, 19 June 2020, https://www.frontiersin.org/articles/10.3389/fimmu.2020.01451/full

176 Kevin Damasio, 'Oxford vaccine enters final phase of COVID-19 trials. Here's what happens now.' 28 July 2020, https://www.nationalgeographic.co.uk/science-and-technology/2020/07/oxford-vaccine-enters-final-phase-of-covid-19-trials-heres-what

177 University of Oxford, 'Oxford COVID-19 vaccine to begin phase II/III human trials', 22 May 2020, https://www.ox.ac.uk/news/2020-05-22-oxford-covid-19-vaccine-begin-phase-iiiii-human-trials

178 ABC News, 'Oxford coronavirus vaccine trial on hold over 'potentially unexplained illness', AstraZeneca says', 9 September 2020, https://www.abc.net.au/news/2020-09-09/coronavirus-vaccine-on-hold-patient-adverse-illness-astrazeneca/12643812

179 AstraZeneca, 'COVID-19 vaccine AZD1222 clinical trials resumed in the UK', press release, 12 September 2020, https://www.astrazeneca.com/media-centre/press-releases/2020/covid-19-vaccine-azd1222-clinical-trials-resumed-in-the-uk.html

180 Oxford Biomedical Research Centre, 'Oxford COVID-19 vaccine begins human trial stage', 23 April 2020, https://oxfordbrc.nihr.ac.uk/oxford-covid-19-vaccine-begins-human-trial-stage/

181 Jade Gailberger, 'Clinical trial pause will not delay Oxford University vaccine', The Weekend Australian, 10 September 2020, https://www.theaustralian.com.au/news/latest-news/clinical-trial-pause-will-not-delay-oxford-university-vaccine/news-story/698421ec536535039eb281bb0aed3961

182 Sir John Bell, Professor, 'These vaccines are unlikely to "completely sterilize" a population. Professor Sir John Bell, SAGE', 29 November 2020, https://www.youtube.com/watch?v=IMAkFKprzRQ and https://foreignaffairsintelligencecouncil.wordpress.com/2020/12/13/oxford-designer-of-covid-vaccine-admits-vaccine-will-only-sterilize-70-per-cent-of-the-population/

183 Australian National Review, 'Head of Pfizer Research: Covid Vaccine is Female Sterilization', December 2020, https://australiannationalreview.com/health/head-of-pfizer-research-covid-vaccine-is-female-sterilization/ Video available at https://www.bitchute.com/video/JJtToV4FuxQ6/

184 Rob Harris, 'Australia COVID vaccine terminated due to HIV 'false positives'', The Sydney Morning Herald, 11 December 2020, https://www.smh.com. au/politics/federal/australian-covid-vaccine-terminated-due-to-hiv-false-positives-20201210-p56mju.html

185 Kerry A. Dolan, 'Bill And Melinda Gates Are Giving Another $70 Million For Covid Vaccines', Forbes, 12 November 2020, https://www.forbes.com/sites/kerryadolan/2020/11/12/bill-and-melinda-gates-are-giving-70-million-more-for-covid-vaccines/?sh=442b036429f8

186 Bill Gates, 'Bill Gates – Normalcy Only Returns After Global Vaccination', 18 April 2020, https://www.youtube.com/watch?v=bXUcBrmNNwM

187 Robert F. Kennedy, Jr., 'New Docs: NIH Owns half of Moderna vaccine', 7 July 2020, https://childrenshealthdefense.org/news/new-docs-nih-owns-half-of-moderna-vaccine/

188 Alex Bruce, 'Trump medical advisor Dr Anthony Fauci owns patent for new Covid vaccine', Cairns News, 7 May 2020, https://cairnsnews.org/2020/05/07/trump-medical-advisor-dr-anthony-fauci-owns-patent-for-new-covid-vaccine/

189 Centers for Disease Control and Prevention, 'Vaccine Effectiveness: How Well Do the Flu Vaccines Work?' n/d, https://www.cdc.gov/flu/vaccines-work/vaccineeffect.htm

190 July Mikovits, PhD, and Joseph Mercola, M.D., 'SARS-CoV-2-Interview with Judy Mikovits', 4 May 2020, https://www.youtube.com/watch?v=eSgN8ONNKVs

191 Children's Health Defense Team, 'Fauci: Steering the Pandemic Narrative Toward Vaccine "Solutions" Is Nothing New', 11 June 2020, https://childrenshealthdefense.org/news/fauci-steering-the-pandemic-narrative-toward-vaccine-solutions-is-nothing-new/

192 The Associated Press, 'More polio cases now caused by vaccine than by wild virus', 26 November 2019, https://abcnews.go.com/Health/wireStory/polio-cases-now-caused-vaccine-wild-virus-67287290

193 Nicola P Klein, in 'Licensed pertussis vaccines in the United States. History and current state', 6 November 2014, https://pubmed.ncbi.nlm.nih.gov/25483496/

194 Robert F. Kennedy, Jr., 'The Bill Gates Effect: WHO's DTP Vaccine Killed More Children in Africa Than the Diseases it Targeted', 23 April 2020, https://childrenshealthdefense.org/news/the-bill-gates-effect-whos-dtp-vaccine-kills-more-children-in-africa-than-the-diseases-it-targets/

195 Soren Wengel Morgensen, et. al., 'The Introduction of Diphtheria-Tetanus-Pertussis and Oral Polio Vaccine Among Young Infants in an Urban African Community: A Natural Experiment', The Lancet, 31 January 2017, https://www.thelancet.com/journals/ebiom/article/PIIS2352-3964(17)30046-4/fulltext

196 Yale University, 'COVID-19 Messaging, Part 1', 7 July 2020, https://clinicaltrials.gov/ct2/show/NCT04460703

197 Peter Breggin, M.D., COVID-19 & Public Health Totalitarianism: Untoward Effects on Individuals, Institutions and Society, 30 August 2020, https://breggin.com/coronavirus/NEW-COVID-19-LEGAL-REPORT.pdf

198 American Society for Pharmacology and Experimental Theraputics 2002, 'Science for the Common Good', Molecular Interventions, Vol. 2 No. 1 17–21, doi 10.1124/mi.2.1.17, February 2002, https://triggered.edina.clockss.org/ServeContent?rft_id=info:doi/10.1124/mi.2.1.17

199 Tenders Electronic Daily, 'Supplies - 506291-2020', 23 October 2020, https://ted.europa.eu/udl?uri=TED:NOTICE:506291-2020:TEXT:EN:HTML

200 Dr Karina Reiss & Dr Sucharit Bhakdi, Corona False Alarm? Facts and Figures, Chelsea Green Publishing, London, UK, 2020, https://www.satrakshita.com/Books/Corona_False_Alarm.pdf

201 CDC, 'COVIDView: Key Updates for Week 51, ending December 19, 2020', updated 28 December 2020, https://www.cdc.gov/coronavirus/2019-ncov/covid-data/covidview/index.html

202 University of Cambridge, 'Research team working toward vaccine against COVID-19', Medical Xpress, 18 March 2020, https://medicalxpress.com/news/2020-03-team-vaccine-covid-.html

203 Dr Alan Finkel, Rapid Research Information Forum: The most promising vaccines for COVID-19, 10 May 2020, https://www.chiefscientist.gov.au/sites/default/files/2020-05/rrif-covid19-promising-vaccines.pdf

204 Catherine J Anderson, et al., 'Impact of Obesity and Metabolic Syndrome on Immunity', Advances in Nutrition, 15 January 2016, https://pubmed.ncbi.nlm.nih.gov/26773015/

205 Harvard Medical School 'How to boost your immune system', Harvard Health Publishing, 6 April 2020, https://www.health.harvard.edu/staying-healthy/how-to-boost-your-immune-system

206 Richard Franki, 'Almost 90% of COVID-19 admissions involve comorbidities', 10 April 2020, https://www.mdedge.com/dermatology/article/220575/coronavirus-updates/almost-90-covid-19-admissions-involve-comorbidities?sso=true

207 Paul Zimmet, PhD, 'Diabesity—The Biggest Epidemic in Human History', Medscape General Medicine, 20 August 2007, https://www.ncbi.nlm.nih.gov/pmc/articles/PMC2100115/

208 Mark Hyman, M.D., 'Nutrition Basics for Everyone', n/d, https://drhyman.com/wp-content/uploads/hyman-downloads/Nutrition%20Basics%20For%20Everyone%20Cheat%20Sheet.pdf

209 Kris Gunnars, 'Mediterranean Diet 101: A Meal Plan and Beginner's Guide', 24 July 2018, https://www.healthline.com/nutrition/mediterranean-diet-meal-plan

210 Husam Dabbagh-Bazarbachi, et al. 'Zinc ionophore activity of quercetin and epigallocatechin-gallate: From Hepa 1-6 Cells to a Liposome Model', Journal of agricultural and food chemistry, 13 August 2014, https://pubmed.ncbi.nlm.nih.gov/25050823/

211 Yejin Kim, 'Vitamin C Is an Essential Factor on the Anti-viral Immune Responses Through the Production of Interferon–a/b at the Initial Stage of Influenza A Virus (H3N2) Infection', Immune Network, 13 April 2013, https://pubmed.ncbi.nlm.nih.gov/23700397/

212 University of Iowa Health Care, 'Why high dose vitamin C kills cancer cells', 9 January 2017, https://www.sciencedaily.com/releases/2017/01/170109134014.htm

213 Michael J Gonzalez, et al., 'High Dose Vitamin C and Influenza: A Case Report', International Society for Orthomolecular Medicine, June 2018, https://isom.ca/article/high-dose-vitamin-c-influenza-case-report/

214 Dr Thomas Levy, 'How to effectively treat viral infections, including Ebola and Zika', 27 February 2016, https://www.peakenergy.com/articles/nh20160227/How-to-effectively-treat-viral-infections-including-Ebola-and-Zika

215 National Health and Medical Research Council, 'Vitamin C', 23 January 2017, https://www.nrv.gov.au/nutrients/vitamin-c

216 Joseph Mercola, M.D., 'How Vitamin C and Magnesium Helps Reverse Disease and Treat Viral Infections', 13 April 2020, https://www.lewrockwell.com/2020/04/joseph-mercola/how-vitamin-c-and-magnesium-helps-reverse-disease-and-treat-viral-infections/

217 Jeffrey Dach, M.D., 'Vitamin C Saves Dying Man', 21 July 2013, https://jeffreydachmd.com/vitamin-c-saves-dying-man/

218 'Proof Vitamin C Miracle Cure? News 60 Minutes', 27 November 2015, https://www.youtube.com/watch?v=Y3VJVScIyD4

219 Ruben Manuel Luciano Colunga Blancatelli, et al., 'Quercetin and Vitamin C: An Experimental, Synergistic Therapy for the Prevention and Treatment of SARS-CoV-2 Related Disease (COVID-19)', Frontiers in Immunology, 19 June 2020, https://www.frontiersin.org/articles/10.3389/fimmu.2020.01451/full

220 Husam Dabbagh-Bazarbachi, et al., 'Zinc ionophore activity of quercetin and epigallocatechin-gallate: from Hepa 1-6 Cells to a liposome model', Journal of agricultural and food chemistry, 13 August 2014, https://pubmed.ncbi.nlm.nih.gov/25050823/

221 Ling Yi, 'Small molecules blocking the entry of severe acute respiratory syndrome coronavirus into host cells', Journal of virology, October 2004, https://pubmed.ncbi.nlm.nih.gov/15452254/

222 Rehan Mehta, 'Vitamin D Deficiency: A New Pandemic', Frontiers, 11 November 2019, https://frontiersmag.wustl.edu/2019/11/11/vitamin-d-deficiency-a-new-pandemic/

223 Joseph Mercola, M.D., 'Vitamin D Cuts SARS-CoV-2 Infection Rate by Half', 28 September 2020, https://articles.mercola.com/sites/articles/archive/2020/09/28/coronavirus-infection-rate-vitamin-d.aspx

224 Avik Roy, in 'Most Important Coronavirus Statistic: 42% of U.S. Deaths are From 0.6% Of The Population', Forbes, 26 May 2020, https://www.forbes.com/sites/theapothecary/2020/05/26/nursing-homes-assisted-living-facilities-0-6-of-the-u-s-population-43-of-u-s-covid-19-deaths/?sh=ce0c92f74cdb

225 James Massola, 'The world's next coronavirus hotspot is emerging next door', The Sydney Morning Herald, 19 June 2020, https://www.smh.com.au/world/asia/the-world-s-next-coronavirus-hotspot-is-emerging-next-door-20200619-p5549q.html

226 Jo Nova, 'Indonesian study: Low Vitamin D patients ten times more likely to die of Coronavirus', n/d, https://joannenova.com.au/2020/05/indonesian-study-low-vitamin-d-patients-ten-times-more-likely-to-die-of-coronavirus/

227 Jose L. Hernandez, et al., 'Vitamin D Status in Hospitalized Patients with SARS-CoV-2 Infection', The Journal of Clinical Endocrinology & Metabolism, 27 October 2020, https://academic.oup.com/jcem/advance-article/doi/10.1210/clinem/dgaa733/5934827

228 Osteoporosis Australia Medical & Scientific Advisory Committee, 'Vitamin D', n/d, https://osteoporosis.org.au/vitamin-d

229 Joseph Mercola, M.D., 'Your Vitamin D Level Must Reach 60 ng/m/L Before the Second Wave', 1 June 2020, https://articles.mercola.com/sites/articles/archive/2020/06/01/vitamin-d-level-to-reach-before-covid-19-second-wave.aspx

230 JL Buttriss & SA Lanham-New, 'Is a vitamin D fortification strategy needed?' National Center for Biotechnology Information, 18 May 2020, https://www.ncbi.nlm.nih.gov/pmc/articles/PMC7276911/

231 Joseph Mercola, M.D., 'Vitamin D Cuts SARS-CoV-2 Infection Rate by Half,' 28 September 2020, https://articles.mercola.com/sites/articles/archive/2020/09/28/coronavirus-infection-rate-vitamin-d.aspx

232 William B. Grant, PhD, et al., Stealth Strategies to Stop COVID Cold, n/d, https://www.stopcovidcold.com/cmstemplates/stopcovidcold/assets/stop%20covid%20cold.pdf

233 Dr Josh Axe, '7 Signs of Zinc Deficiency and the Best Foods to Reverse It!' 24 May 2019, https://draxe.com/nutrition/zinc-deficiency/

234 The Analyst, 'Pyroluria', n/d, https://www.diagnose-me.com/symptoms-of/pyroluria.php

235 Dr Jockers, 'Pyroluria: The Most Common Unknown Disorder', n/d, https://drjockers.com/pyroluria-common-unknown-disorder/

236 'Immune Function and Micronutrient Requirements Change over the Life Course', Nutrients, October 2018, https://pubmed.ncbi.nlm.nih.gov/30336639/

237 Husam Dabbagh-Bazarbachi, et al., 'Zinc Ionophore Activity of quercetin and epigallocatechin-gallate: From Hepa 1-6 cells to a Liposome Model', Journal of agricultural and food chemistry, August 2014, https://pubmed.ncbi.nlm.nih.gov/25050823/

238 Mohammad Tariqur Rahman & Syed Zahir Idid, 'Can Zn Be a Critical Element in COVID-19 Treatment?' 26 May 2020, https://pubmed.ncbi.nlm.nih.gov/32458149/

239 David Brownstein, M.D., et al., 'A Novel Approach to Treating COVID-19 Using Nutritional and Oxidative Therapies', Science, Public Health Policy, and the Law, July 2020, https://ozonewithoutborders.ngo/wp-content/uploads/2020/07/Novel-Approach-to-Covid-19.pdf

240 Front Line COVID-19 Critical Care Alliance, 'Prophylaxis and Treatment Protocols for COVID-19', updated January 2021, https://covid19criticalcare.com/

241 Front Line COVID-19 Critical Care Alliance, 'MATH+ Hospital Treatment Protocol for COVID-19', n/d, https://covid19criticalcare.com/math-hospital-treatment/

242 Front Line COVID-19 Critical Care Alliance, 'Prophylaxis and Treatment Protocols for COVID-19', n/d, https://covid19criticalcare.com/

243 COVID.US.ORG, 'The MATH+ Protocol for Prevention and Treatment of Covid-19', 24 June 2020 (updated 12 December 2020), https://covid.us.org/2020/06/24/the-math-protocol-for-prevention-and-treatment-of-covid-19/

244 Stop COVID Cold, 'Proven, Natural, Safe, Effective and Inexpensive Ways to Enhance Your Immune System', n/d, https://www.stopcovidcold.com/

245 Thomas E. Levy, M.D., J.D., 'COVID-19: How can I cure thee? Let me count the ways', 18 July 2020, http://www.orthomolecular.org/resources/omns/v16n37.shtml

246 Kevin Hartnett, 'The Tricky Math of Herd Immunity for COVID-19', 30 June 2020, https://www.quantamagazine.org/the-tricky-math-of-covid-19-herd-immunity-20200630/

247 Shikha Garg, M.D., et al., 'Hospitalization Rates and Characteristics of Patients Hospitalized with Laboratory-Confirmed Coronavirus Disease 2019—COVID-NET, 14 States, March 1-30, 2020', 17 April 2020, https://www.cdc.gov/mmwr/volumes/69/wr/mm6915e3.htm

248 Raymond Obomsawin, PhD., 'Immunization Graphs: Natural Infectious Disease Declines; Immunization Effectiveness; and Immunization Dangers', December 2009, http://whale.to/vaccine/ImmunizationGraphs-RO2009.pdf

249 Greg Beattie, 'Vaccination Dilemma: The vaccine effort in historical perspective', n/d, https://vaccinationdilemma.com/historical-death-rates-diseases-vaccination-html/

250 David Hogberg, 'Will the US achieve COVID-19 herd immunity before a vaccine?' Washington Examiner, 3 September 2020, https://www.washingtonexaminer.com/news/will-the-us-achieve-covid-19-herd-immunity-before-a-vaccine

251 Carl O'Donnell, 'Fauci warns COVID-19 vaccine may be only partially effective, public health measures still needed', Reuters, 8 August 2020, https://www.reuters.com/article/us-health-coronavirus-fauci-vaccine-idUSKCN2532YX

252 Yoni Heiser, 'Dr. Fauci just gave us some pretty scary news about coronavirus vaccines', 9 August 2020, https://bgr.com/2020/08/09/coronavirus-vaccine-effective-fauci-50-percent/

253 Senator Marise Payne, 'Australia and the world in the time of COVID-19', 16 June 2020, https://www.foreignminister.gov.au/minister/marise-payne/speech/australia-and-world-time-covid-19

254 Australian Government Department of Health, 'Eliminating COVID-19 a false hope', 16 July 2020, https://www.health.gov.au/news/eliminating-covid-19-a-false-hope

255 Ben Knight, 'Has the coronavirus pandemic proved that homelessness is solvable?' ABC News, 8 June 2020, https://www.abc.net.au/news/2020-06-08/housing-homeless-in-pandemic-has-worked-lets-make-it-permanent/12330442

256 Tom McIlroy, 'Australia 'ripe for economic reform': NSW Premier', Financial Review, 17 May 2020, https://www.afr.com/politics/federal/australia-ripe-for-economic-reform-nsw-premier-20200517-p54tpz

257 Bruce Lipton, 'Bruce Lipton Explains How Thoughts Cause Disease in the Body', 26 August 2019, https://www.fearlessmotivation.com/2019/08/26/bruce-lipton-explains-how-thoughts-cause-disease-in-the-body/

258 Australian Human Rights Commission, 'Universal Declaration of Human Rights – Human rights at your fingertips', 14 December 2012, https://humanrights.gov.au/our-work/commission-general/universal-declaration-human-rights-human-rights-your-fingertips-human

259 Joseph Mercola, M.D., 'Emotional Freedom Techniques (EFT) Demonstration', 11 May 2011, https://www.youtube.com/watch?v=IWu3rSEddZI

260 Joseph Mercola, M.D., 'EFT Helps Improve Your Health By Freeing Yourself from Stress', 25 April 2013, https://articles.mercola.com/sites/articles/archive/2013/04/25/eft-relieves-stress.aspx

261 Alexandra Carlton, 'The Terrifying Rise Of Domestic Violence In Isolation: Inside our other deadly pandemic', 14 May 2020, https://www.marieclaire.com.au/domestic-violence-isolation-covid-19

262 Alex Crowe, 'Child abuse websites crash during coronavirus lockdowns', The Canberra Times, 7 June 2020, https://www.canberratimes.com.au/story/6783641/child-abuse-websites-crash-during-coronavirus-lockdowns/

263 Melissa L. Davey, 'Child abuse predator 'handbook' lists ways to target children during coronavirus lockdown', 14 May 2020, https://www.theguardian.com/society/2020/may/14/child-abuse-predator-handbook-lists-ways-to-target-children-during-coronavirus-lockdown

264 Meagan Dillon, 'Child exploitation websites 'crashing' during coronavirus amid sharp rise in reported abuse', ABC News, 20 May 2020, https://www.abc.net.au/news/2020-05-20/afp-concerned-by-child-exploitation-spike-amid-coronavirus/12265544

265 Tammy Mills, 'New reports of family violence spike in COVID-19 lockdown, study finds', The Age, 8 June 2020, https://www.theage.com.au/national/victoria/new-reports-of-family-violence-spike-in-covid-19-lockdown-study-finds-20200607-p55096.html

266 Shannon Molloy, 'The silent death toll of COVID-19 revealed: Huge 25 per cent jump in suicides each year', 25 July 2020, https://www.news.com.au/lifestyle/health/health-problems/the-silent-death-toll-of-covid19-revealed-huge-25-per-cent-jump-in-suicides-each-year/news-story/b4154626a16c9cc25c3b79b7880041ef

267 Kim Trengove, 'Suicide deaths could surge post COVID-19', Australian Men's Health Forum, n/d, https://www.amhf.org.au/suicide_deaths_could_surge_post_covid_19

268 Kim Trengove, 'Social isolation increases male suicide risk says AMHF', Australian Men's Health Forum, n/d, https://www.amhf.org.au/social_isolation_increases_male_suicide_risk_says_amhf

269 Kimberley Drake, 'COVID-19: Quicker recovery may indicate long-term immunity', Medical News Today, 6 November 2020, https://www.medicalnewstoday.com/articles/covid-19-quicker-recovery-may-indicate-long-term-immunity

270 Pam Belluck, 'Here's What Recovery From Covid-19 Looks Like for Many Survivors', The New York Times, 1 July 2020, https://www.nytimes.com/2020/07/01/health/coronavirus-recovery-survivors.html

271 The World Bank, 'The Global Economic Outlook During the COVID-19 Pandemic: A Changed World', 8 June 2020, https://www.worldbank.org/en/news/feature/2020/06/08/the-global-economic-outlook-during-the-covid-19-pandemic-a-changed-world

272 Australian Bureau of Statistics, 'Business Indicators, Business Impacts of COVID-19', 30 July 2020, https://www.abs.gov.au/statistics/economy/business-indicators/business-indicators-business-impacts-covid-19/jul-2020

273 Helen Regan and Angus Watson, 'Qantas boss says passengers will need to be vaccinated for international flights', 24 November 2020, https://edition.cnn.com/travel/article/qantas-coronavirus-vaccination-intl-hnk-scli/index.html

274 Tony Robbins, 'Where Focus Goes, Energy Flows: Create a vision for your business and your life', n/d, https://www.tonyrobbins.com/career-business/where-focus-goes-energy-flows/

275 Lao Tzu (with commentary by Rory B Mackay), Tao Te Ching, Blue Star Publishing, 19 May 2007, https://www.booktopia.com.au/tao-te-ching-new-edition-with-commentary--lao-tzu/book/9780993267550.html

276 Centers for Disease Control and Prevention, 'Ebola Virus Distribution Map: Case of Ebola Virus Disease in Africa since 1996', reviewed 1 December 2020, https://www.cdc.gov/vhf/ebola/history/distribution-map.html

277 Worldometer, 'COVID-19 Coronavirus Pandemic', updated daily, https://www.worldometers.info/coronavirus/

278 Evan Andrews, 'Why Was It Called the Spanish Flu?' 12 January 2016 (updated 27 March, 2020), https://www.history.com/news/why-was-it-called-the-spanish-flu

279 Rebecca Forgasz, 'Coronavirus: What past pandemics teach us about COVID-19', 10 June 2020, https://lens.monash.edu/@politics-society/2020/06/10/1380621/coronavirus-what-can-past-pandemics-teach-us-about-covid-19

280 Milton J. Rosenau, 'Experiments to Determine Mode of Spread of Influenza', Journal of the American Medical Association (JAMA), 2 August 2019, https://zenodo.org/record/1505669

281 Today, 'How do pandemics end?' 17 May 2020, https://www.todayonline.com/world/how-do-pandemics-end

282 Gina Kolata, 'How Pandemics End', 14 May 2020, https://www.nytimes.com/2020/05/10/health/coronavirus-plague-pandemic-history.html

283 Sherryn Groch, 'Could Australia eliminate COVID-19 like NZ and how would it work?' The Sydney Morning Herald, 22 July 2020, https://www.smh.com.au/national/could-we-eliminate-covid-19-in-australia-and-how-would-it-work-20200721-p55e0k.html

284 Carolyn Whitzman, 'Silver Lining: Could COVID-19 lead to a better future?' The Conversation, 25 March 2020, https://theconversation.com/silver-lining-could-covid-19-lead-to-a-better-future-134204

285 Stephen Dowling, 'Coronavirus: What can we learn from the Spanish flu?' 3 March 2020, https://www.bbc.com/future/article/20200302-coronavirus-what-can-we-learn-from-the-spanish-flu

286 American Journal of Public Health, Vol. 8 Issue 10, pp. 787–788, Doi: 10.2105/AJPH.8.10.787, 'Weapons Against Influenza.', Editorial, 1 October 1918, https://ajph.aphapublications.org/doi/pdf/10.2105/AJPH.8.10.787

287 Richard Hobday, 'Coronavirus and the Sun: A Lesson from the 1918 Influenza Pandemic', 10 March 2020, https://medium.com/@ra.hobday/coronavirus-and-the-sun-a-lesson-from-the-1918-influenza-pandemic-509151dc8065

288 Richard J. Hobday, PhD., and John W. Cason, PhD., 'The Open-Air Treatment of Pandemic Influenza', American Journal of Public Health, 20 September 2011, https://ajph.aphapublications.org/doi/full/10.2105/AJPH.2008.134627

289 Thomas F. Sheridan, 'Pandemics and politics: Lessons the HIV/AIDS crisis', The Hill, 25 April 2020, https://thehill.com/opinion/healthcare/494565-pandemics-and-politics-lessons-from-the-hiv-aids-crisis

290 Justin Denholm, 'What we've learnt from four other pandemics throughout history', 17 April 2020, https://www.sbs.com.au/news/what-we-ve-learned-from-four-other-pandemics-throughout-history

291 Wikipedia, 'Work for the Dole', n/d, https://en.wikipedia.org/wiki/Work_for_the_Dole

292 Avik Roy, 'Most Important Coronavirus Statistic: 42% of US deaths are from 0.6% of the population', Forbes, 26 May 2020, https://www.forbes.com/sites/theapothecary/2020/05/26/nursing-homes-assisted-living-facilities-0-6-of-the-u-s-population-43-of-u-s-covid-19-deaths/?sh=74025bd674cd

293 J. MacLaughlin and M.F. Holick, 'Aging Decreases the Capacity of Human Skin to Produce Vitamin D3.', The Journal of Clinical Investigation, October 1985, https://www.ncbi.nlm.nih.gov/pmc/articles/PMC424123/

294 Amanda Lee, 'What is China's social credit system and why is it controversial?' The South China Morning Post, 9 August 2020, https://www.scmp.com/economy/china-economy/article/3096090/what-chinas-social-credit-system-and-why-it-controversial

295 Xinyuan Wang, 'Hundreds of Chinese citizens told me what they thought about the controversial social credit system', The Conversation, 17 December 2019, https://theconversation.com/hundreds-of-chinese-citizens-told-me-what-they-thought-about-the-controversial-social-credit-system-127467

296 Ellen Brown, 'From lockdown to Police State: The "Great Reset" Rolls Out', Global Research, 23 August 2020, https://www.globalresearch.ca/lockdown-police-state-great-reset-rolls-out/5721845

297 Antonia do Carmo Barriga, et al., 'The COVID-19 pandemic: Yet another catalyst for governmental mass surveillance?' Science Direct Social Sciences & Humanities Open, 2020, https://www.sciencedirect.com/science/article/pii/S2590291120300851

298 Michael Ashley, 'A Tale Of Two Cities In The Age Of COVID-19', Forbes, 21 April 2020, https://www.forbes.com/sites/cognitiveworld/2020/04/21/a-tale-of-two-cities-in-the-age-of-covid-19/?sh=e4d62536aeb8

299 Kevin Nguyen, 'The QR code has turned COVID-19 check-ins into a golden opportunity for marketing and data companies', ABC News, 2 November 2020, https://www.abc.net.au/news/2020-10-31/covid-19-check-in-data-using-qr-codes-raises-privacy-concerns/12823432

300 Joe Waters, 'Security Risks that Come with Use of QR Codes', n/d, https://www.dummies.com/business/marketing/social-media-marketing/security-risks-that-come-with-use-of-qr-codes/

301 Alex Hern, 'Cambridge Analytica: how did it turn clicks into votes?' 6 May 2020, https://www.theguardian.com/news/2018/may/06/cambridge-analytica-how-turn-clicks-into-votes-christopher-wylie

302 Vyacheslav Polonski, 'How artificial intelligence conquered democracy', 8 August 2020, https://theconversation.com/how-artificial-intelligence-conquered-democracy-77675

303 Gregory C. Allen, 'Putin and Musk are right: Whoever masters AI will run the world', 5 September 2017, https://edition.cnn.com/2017/09/05/opinions/russia-weaponize-ai-opinion-allen/index.html

304 Profusa, Inc., 'Profusa and Partners Receive DARPA Award to Speed Detection of Disease Outbreaks', 8 August 2019, https://www.prnewswire.com/news-releases/profusa-and-partners-receive-darpa-award-to-speed-detection-of-disease-outbreaks-300898518.html

305 Makia Freeman, 'Hydrogel Biosensor: Implantable Nanotech to be Used in COVID Vaccines?' 2 September 2020, https://thefreedomarticles.com/hydrogel-biosensor-darpa-gates-implantable-nanotech-covid-vaccine/

306 Joseph Mercola, M.D., 'Injectable Biochip for SARS-CoV-2 Detection Near FDA Approval', 17 September 2020, https://www.lewrockwell.com/2020/09/joseph-mercola/injectable-biochip-for-sars-cov-2-detection-near-fda-approval/

307 Dr David Martin, https://www.davidmartin.world/about/

308 'Dr David Martin and Judy Mikovits Explain why the mRNA Vaccine is not a Vaccine', BitChute, 16 January 2021, https://www.bitchute.com/video/2ibqm6gSBnzA/

309 Adam Keiper, 'The Nanotechnology Revolution', The New Atlantis, 2003, https://www.thenewatlantis.com/publications/the-nanotechnology-revolution

310 Ben Gilbert, 'Elon Musk says he's terrified of AI taking over the world and most scared of Google's DeepMind AI project', Business Insider Australia, 28 July 2020, https://www.businessinsider.com.au/elon-musk-maureen-dowd-ai-google-deepmind-wargames-2020-7

311 Joseph Mercola, M.D., 'Why Lockdowns Don't Work and Hurt the Most Vulnerable', 30 December 2020, https://articles.mercola.com/sites/articles/archive/2020/12/30/lockdowns-do-not-work.aspx

312 Paul Salmon, et al., 'To protect us from the risks of advanced artificial intelligence, we need to act now', The Conversation, 25 January 2019, https://theconversation.com/to-protect-us-from-the-risks-of-advanced-artificial-intelligence-we-need-to-act-now-107615

313 Hassaan Janjua, et al., 'Trusted Operations on Sensor Data', Sensors (Basel), 27 April 2018, https://www.ncbi.nlm.nih.gov/pmc/articles/PMC5982508/

314 Tracy Brower, 'What Hard Times Teach Us: 5 Pandemic-Inspired Lessons That Will Make You Better For The Long Term', Forbes, 19 April 2020, https://www.forbes.com/sites/tracybrower/2020/04/19/what-hard-times-teach-us-5-pandemic-inspired-lessons-that-will-make-you-better-for-the-long-term/?sh=514f795819c9

315 P.S. Jayaramu, 'COVID-19 and the emerging International Balance of Power', Mainstream, 24 October 2020, https://www.mainstreamweekly.net/article10037.html

316 Kevin Rudd, 'The Coming Post-COVID Anarchy', Foreign Affairs, 6 May 2020, https://www.foreignaffairs.com/articles/united-states/2020-05-06/coming-post-covid-anarchy

317 The Johns Hopkins News-Letter, 'A closer look at U.S. deaths due to COVID-19', 22 November 2020, https://corona-transition.org/IMG/pdf/a_closer_look_at_u.s._deaths_due_to_covid-19_-_the_johns_hopkins_news-letter.pdf

About the Author

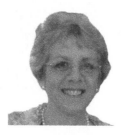

Growing up on a farm in remote New South Wales taught Margaret the value of critical thinking and creative learning from a young age, which became her accepted norm. Tragic experiences during her life have taught her valuable coping skills where she was able to build resilience and learn the importance of kindness, empathy and compassion. Margaret has a passionate interest in health, social justice and ethics and its these values that motivated her to write this book.

Margaret Stevenson (B.SocSc) (Cert.Nut) is an Australian writer of transformational non-fiction. She published a family history book in 2003 and was awarded first place in the Country Women's Association of New South Wales *Garry Prize Short Story Competition* in 2017 and third place in the same competition in 2018. She has held the positions of publicity officer and secretary for several volunteer organisations over many years. Margaret lives in rural New South Wales and enjoys arts, crafts, family life and community.

CPSIA information can be obtained
at www.ICGtesting.com
Printed in the USA
LVHW032302230421
685383LV00002B/249